The Itinerary of a Breakfast

Breakfast

The Stages of Digestion; Gastro-Intestinal Care and Nutrition in the Eating of a Healthy Morning Meal

By John Harvey Kellogg

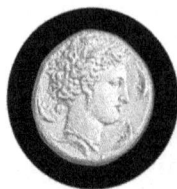

PANTIANOS
CLASSICS

Published by Pantianos Classics

ISBN-13: 978-1-78987-211-8

First published in 1918

Contents

Preface

Modern medical research has clearly incriminated the colon as the source of more disease and physical suffering than any other organ of the body.

The artificial conditions of civilized life, sedentary habits, concentrated foodstuffs, false modesty, ignorance and neglect of bodily needs, have produced a crippled state of the colon as an almost universal condition among civilized men and women.

Intestinal toxemia or autointoxication is the most universal of all maladies, and the source of autointoxication is the colon with its seething mass of putrefying food residues.

A very special purpose in the mind of the author in the preparation of this little volume has been to combat some of the mischievous errors which are everywhere current in relation to the hygiene of the colon, especially with reference to the sufficiency of one daily evacuation of the food residues. It seems to the author that no one can review the facts here set forth without being convinced that food residues and wastes should be evacuated at least three times a day, or after each meal.

In the chapters, "The Ten Gates," "The House-broken Colon" and "The Crippled Colon," new facts brought forward by modern research and discovery are grouped together in a new way which it is hoped the reader will find interesting as well as informing.

The call for information on the vital question of "waste disposal" is steadily increasing. It is hoped that the additional light which it is believed this volume sheds upon this subject will prove of interest and practical value to every careful reader.

Practical assistance will be found in the author's works, "Colon Hygiene," "Autointoxication," and various other works on food and diet issued by the publishers of this work as well as in the monthly columns of *"Good Health."*

The Food Tube

The food tube, or *prima viae*, as it was termed by the ancients, is a muscular tube through which the food travels a distance of about ten yards in its transit of the body. This journey along the alimentary canal, however, is not at all comparable to the passage of water or other liquid along a pipe. The food canal is, in fact, not an open tube into and along which liquids may be poured, like a water pipe or a rubber tube, but a soft, flexible, ever-changing hollow muscle which adapts its size to its contents and tightly grasps and manipulates them and continually pushes them along by means of contraction waves which travel rhythmically from above downward so long as there is anything present in the tube, either solid, liquid, or gaseous.

When solids or liquids leave the mouth, then, they do not drop through a hollow tube into our interiors, but are seized or grasped by the muscular walls of the food tube and are forcibly carried on from point to point by purposive and rhythmical automatic muscular movements.

The mucous lining of the tube is so sensitive that the smallest particles are noticed and dealt with. This is well shown in the mouth. A minute particle, as a

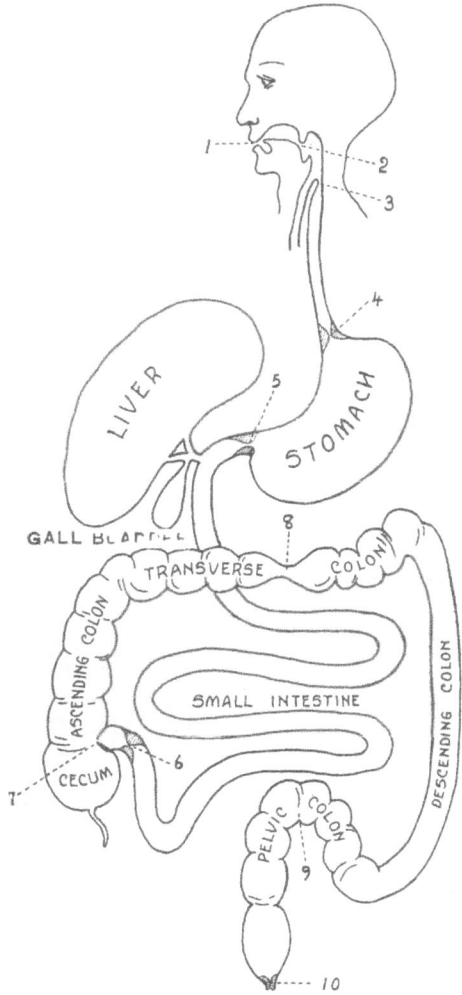

Diagram of Food Tube, Showing the Ten Gates which control the movement of food along the canal. 1, Mouth; 2, Fauces; 3, Entrance to Oesophagus; 4, Cardiac Orifice of Stomach; 5, Pylorus; 6, Ileocecal Sphincter; 7, Ileocecal Valve; 8, Keith's Node, seat of reverse peristalsis; 9, Pelvic Colon; 10, Anus.

seed or flake of bran, will keep the tongue busy until it has been dislodged and disposed of. A very small particle lodged far back in the throat will pro-

duce gagging, coughing or other expulsive efforts until swallowed or rejected.

This same sensitiveness to contacts exists all the way along the food tube
from entrance to exit, although after the food is swallowed, we are not, when
in health, conscious of the automatic efforts by which they are moved along.

When the tube contents are bulky, distending or stretching its muscular
walls, these contraction waves, so-called peristaltic waves, are vigorous and
may even become painfully violent as in colic. When no food has been taken
for twelve hours or more, the intestine is inactive. During fasting there is
practically no intestinal activity.

The eminent English anatomist Keith has shown that the movements of the
stomach and intestines are controlled by a mechanism much the same as that
which controls the heart.

His "Serpent"

The intestinal movements are, moreover, directed with such evident purpose and precision as almost to suggest that the food tube is an independent
and intelligent creature, possessing its own brain and will and ever perform-
ing its functions as a faithful body-servant.

The movements of the intestine are so much like those which one sees executed by a moving snake, that a noted writer very naturally referred to his
food tube as his "serpent," and certain movements of the colon are referred
to in medical literature as snakelike movements.

When the nerves of an arm, a leg, or almost any other organ of the body,
are severed, so that connection with the brain or spinal cord is cut off, the
organ is at once paralyzed. It is as powerless to act as though it were actually
separated from the body. This is by no means the case with the food canal.
An experiment made by Professor Roger, of Paris, will illustrate this. A stick
pin was placed in the intestine of an animal, the point being directed downward. At once a series of most interesting movements began. As the point of
the pin began to penetrate the wall of the intestine, the tissues began to
thicken, thus preventing an immediate puncture.

At the same time, a fold of the intestine pushed up beneath the head of the
pin and pushed it over, so that in a short time the pin was completely reversed, the head being directed downstream in the intestine, and by the contraction of the bowel pushed along until it was discharged from the body.
This wonderful action was seen to take place in the intestine, even after all
the nerves connecting the intestine with the brain had been severed.

In an equally intelligent manner the stomach and intestines deal with the
food, moving it along from point to point as is necessary to perfect the work
of digestion and absorption, retaining it when necessary in various pouches
for special purposes, and even sending it back from one point to another to
meet certain exigencies which may arise. But our habits of eating are so un-
natural, and our neglect of our bodily welfare so great, that in spite of Na-

ture's elaborate precautions and marvelous adaptations, very few persons reach adult age without getting their colons so badly crippled that they are compelled to suffer almost constantly from miseries and inconveniences from which they seek relief in vain through the use of cathartic pills, "salts," mineral waters, and a long list of drugs, every one of which is decidedly injurious and an aggravation of the very conditions it is expected to relieve. Laxative drugs are the most active of all causes of constipation.

Food the Natural Laxative

When food is taken into the stomach, the movements of the tube become very vigorous. Indeed, while the food is still in the mouth and being chewed, and before a morsel has been swallowed, the movements begin, and are four times as vigorous during the taking of a meal as at other times. This is a very excellent reason why constipated persons should eat deliberately, taking ample time at meals and chewing long and well. Food is the natural laxative. The act of eating starts the action of the muscular machinery by means of which first the food and later the food residues are transported along the alimentary canal, and so long as chewing continues new impulses are continually transmitted to the stomach and intestines which quicken the peristaltic movements and activity of the whole digestive machine. The observations of Hirsch, Case and others have shown that the colon contents advance as far during the hour of eating as during four hours just before the meal.

This interesting fact has heretofore received no attention from writers in practical hygiene, although the beneficial influence of eating an orange or an apple at night has long been recognized. This fact is no doubt also the explanation of the beneficial effect of drinking cold water before breakfast and at bedtime.

Stations along the Road

The food tube is like a street in London. Although continuous, it bears different names at different points along its course. Named in their natural order, the several divisions of the alimentary canal are as follows:

The *mouth;* the *fauces;* the *gullet* or *oesophagus;* the *stomach;* the *duodenum,* short upper part of small intestine; *jejunum,* upper part of small intestine below the duodenum; *ileum,* lower half of small intestine; *cecum,* the first part of the colon; *ascending colon,* section of the large intestine extending from cecum to liver; *transverse colon,* middle portion which passes across the abdominal cavity from the liver on the right to the spleen in the left; the *descending colon,* part which lies between the spleen and the left hip bone; iliac colon, the portion lying in the hollow of the left hip bone; the *pelvic colon,* the free loop which connects the iliac colon with the rectum; the *rectum,* the terminal part of the large intestine, normally empty; the *anus,* the exit of the food tube guarded by a circular or sphincter muscle, the anal sphincter; fifteen divisions in all.

Food Principles

The materials of which a breakfast is composed are not homeogenous. Food is made up of a variety of very diverse elements, known as food principles of which there are two groups:

1. *Major food principles,* which constitute the bulk of our foods. These are:

a. Carbohydrates, that is foodstuffs made up of the elements carbon, hydrogen, and oxygen, or really, carbon and water. Starch, sugar, dextrine and the acids of fruits and vegetables make up this class.

b. Fats, hydrocarbons, substances consisting chiefly of carbon and hydrogen. All sorts of edible animal and vegetable fats and oils belong to this class.

c. Proteins, food substances made up of hydrogen, oxygen and carbon, with the addition of nitrogen, sulphur, and phosphorus. White of egg 9 the lean of meat, the curd of milk, and the gluten of wheat are examples of protein.

All of these substances are combustible, and they are burned in the body, but they are not equally useful as fuel. In fact, proteins are hardly to be considered as fuels. When starch and fats burn, the combustion products are simple, odorless and harmless carbon dioxide and water. When protein burns, the products are highly poisonous and foul-smelling gases.

The purpose of protein is to supply material for building and repairing the tissues, the machinery of the body.

These major food principles may be classified then, as (1) *Fuel* food principles — starch, sugar and fats, and (2) *Tissue building* food principles, the proteins.

2. *Minor food principles.*

These are also three in number, viz., salts, cellulose, and vitamines.

The *salts* consist chiefly of lime, soda, potash, magnesia and iron, combined with the principal mineral acids.

Cellulose is found in vegetable food only. It is highly important as a bulk forming element and is necessary to stimulate the food tube to proper activity.

Vitamines are subtle elements in the food which are essential to good nutrition, and in the absence of which various deficiency disorders make their appearance, such as beriberi, scurvy, and probably pellagra and rickets.

Vitamines are easily destroyed by boiling or baking and by long drying. This fact emphasizes the need of a daily and abundant supply of fresh fruit and vegetables which have not been impaired by cooking.

It must also be remembered that vitamines are chiefly found in the outer coverings of seeds and in the germ, and so are not found in fine wheat flour nor polished rice. Vitamines abound in fruit and vegetable juices, especially the juice of the orange. Green leaves (uncooked) such as lettuce, cabbage, and spinach, are rich in vitamines.

The Five Food Laboratories

The crude materials which we eat cannot be used for blood making or tissue building until they have been reduced to simple, homogeneous elements and refined and modified by various chemico-vital processes which take place in the *mouth, stomach, small intestine, liver* and *colon,* each of which is a veritable food laboratory in which most remarkable chemical fluids, the digestive juices, are formed, by which the necessary changes are produced in the several elements of the food.

These changes are absolutely essential to life, and must be complete and efficient or nutrition will fail, strength and energy will depreciate and finally the life processes will cease.

The Mouth Laboratory — The Mill

First in order is the mouth, the mill which grinds the food by thorough mastication.

The chewing of agreeable food starts up the whole digestive machinery. The saliva flows freely, the gastric and other juices likewise begin to flow (appetite juice — Pavlov) and the peristalic waves which move the food along the food tube from one laboratory to another, start in the stomach and travel along the whole thirty feet of the alimentary canal.

The saliva softens the food and also transforms some of the starch into sugar (malt sugar) by the action of a starch-digesting ferment which it contains. The longer the food is chewed the more completely the starch is digested, and the larger the amount of gastric juice produced in the stomach in readiness to digest the food when it arrives.

Proper chewing of the food also serves a useful purpose in regulating the food intake. The thorough tasting of the food permits the nerves of taste to judge the quality of the food and to regulate the intake to suit the needs of the body, a most important function. Hasty eating and overeating go together.

Thorough mastication of the food helps to preserve the teeth by giving them the exercise they need.

Persons who suffer from sour stomach, a condition due to an excess of hydrochloric acid secretion, should chew little, and so should eat soft food that needs little mastication.

The Stomach Laboratory

The action of the saliva continues in the stomach.

The stomach makes a strongly acid fluid, the gastric juice, which breaks up and softens the food by dissolving certain of the proteins; but it does not complete the work, and very little absorption takes place in the stomach. Gastric digestion is a sort of preliminary change in the food by which it is prepared for the action of the digestive fluids of the small intestine.

The Chief Food Laboratory

The small intestine is the great food laboratory of the body. Here the main work of digestion is done. Nearly all the digestible food principles are here completely transformed and prepared for blood and tissue building.

In the small intestine absorption is surprisingly active. There are 5,000,000 villi, the special absorbents of the intestine, each of which, working constantly, absorbs about one ounce of liquid in a life time of sixty years.

The small intestine normally absorbs about six quarts of liquid food stuffs daily. The colon absorbs only 10-20 ounces daily.

The food material which passes through the intestine may be regarded as the soil out of which the body grows. The villi are the rootlets which suck up the nourishment by which the body is developed and maintained.

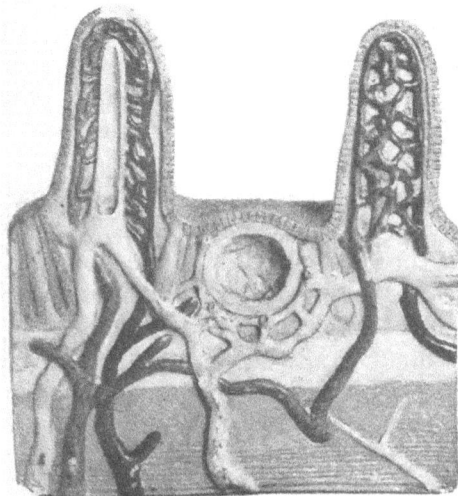

Cross-Section of Villi from the Small Intestine

The Liver Laboratory — The Refinery

Outside the food tube, but directly connected with it, is a wonderful laboratory to which practically all of the food goes after absorption and before entering the general blood current. Here the various products of digestion undergo the final delicate changes needed to prepare them for the various parts which they are to play in the repair and maintenance of the body. In this laboratory more work is done, and a greater variety of work, than is accomplished by any other gland in the body, a fact which is the more surprizing as, from an anatomical standpoint the structure of the liver is very simple, giving no suggestion of the astonishing versatility of its work.

The Waste-Disposal System

One more important laboratory remains to be described, — the colon, the waste-disposal system of the body. By the time the foodstuffs have passed through the twenty-two feet of small intestine, the digestible and absorbable matters have been practically all digested and absorbed.

Out of the pound and a half of water-free digestible food usually eaten daily, only a small fraction is usually found in the material which enters the colon from the small intestine. The colon has little to do but to dispose of the unusable food remnants and of the excretory waste matters which enter the colon from the blood. The food residues contain billions of bacteria, which sometimes constitute more than half of the whole mass of the feces.

The first half of the colon acts as a reducing plant, absorbing a part of the water, by which the bulk of the material to be disposed of is reduced more than one half.

The second half of the colon, the terminal part of the food tube, has no other function than to transmit and eject from the body the waste and poisonous matters which constitute the feces or the stool.

The Normal Intestinal Rhythm — Three Daily Evacuations

Under normal conditions, when all parts of the digestive tube are doing their work efficiently, the colon discharges its contents at least three times a day. The residue of each meal is dismissed after the second following meal. That is, the food residues from the daily breakfast should be discharged by a bowel movement between supper and bedtime.

The following is the order of the food procession for the three daily meals:

Breakfast leaves the stomach and reaches the lower part of the small intestine in four to five hours (see diagram). The vigorous activity set up by the taking of dinner pushes the breakfast residue over into the colon, the middle part of which is reached within nine or ten hours. Between dinner and supper, the breakfast residue slowly works along to the lower end of the colon; and when supper is eaten, the new and vigorous peristaltic waves started in the stomach sweep the dinner residue into the colon, and should carry out of the body the breakfast residue all ready, waiting close to the outlet to be dismissed.

During the night, the breakfast residue works slowly along the colon to the lower end, and the supper residue passes over from the small intestine into the colon. The stimulus of awakening and the effort of rising often produce a bowel movement before breakfast by which the dinner residue is dismissed.

After breakfast, the supper residue is dismissed by the strong peristaltic waves set up by the meal, which should completely empty the colon.

When the colon is thus swept clean of all body wastes and food residues once in twenty-four hours, there is no time for putrefaction, and the stools are free from the loathsome odors of decay which are commonly present. Under such circumstances, the blood remains free from the pollution which must result from the stagnation of food residues which have been retained for many successive days until putrefaction processes have reached a very advanced stage. The liver, lungs, kidneys, and skin are not compelled to act as sewers in attempting to carry off the filth which the colon has failed to dispose of.

So long as the body wastes are disposed of in this prompt and normal manner, the terrible effects which arise from intestinal toxemia or autointoxication are not seen. The skin is clear, the tongue clean, the breath sweet, the appetite keen, the mind active, optimistic and serene, sleep sound and restful, endurance great and resistance high.

Unfortunately, this happy state is seldom met among civilized people who have advanced beyond the age of infancy. The customs of civilized life nearly all tend to render the colon sluggish, and to cripple its function as a waste-disposal system. The flesh-eating habit loads the colon with the remnants of undigested flesh which undergo the same changes which take place in the decaying carcass of a dead animal left to itself. Thus, the body is flooded with the most horrible and loathsome poisons, and the marvel is not that human life is so short and so full of miseries, mental, moral, and physical, but that civilized human beings are able to live at all. The civilized colon with its accumulated residue of five to fifteen meals or more, is a Golgotha of pollution, a veritable Pandora's box of disease.

Modern science has not only taught us how the normal colon should act, but how the diseased colon may be reformed. By a proper diet and proper management, even very obstinate colons may be made to act three times a day. Even colons which have become so badly twisted out of shape by adhesions and kinks, and so paralyzed by overdistension that they cannot be restored by the simple means mentioned may, by the wonderful resources of modern surgery, be made to perform their function in a perfectly satisfactory manner. And thus it may be said safely that every case of constipation, no matter how obstinate, or what its cause, may be substantially relieved.

In other words, the obstacles which bad habits and resulting disease create along the food tube may be removed, so that the delays which produce intestinal toxemia with all its horrible consequences may be prevented and the normal itinerary re-established.

The alimentary canal may be considered as divided into four apartments, in each of which the food is retained for a time to undergo changes which are not only essential to the digestive process, but are necessary to prepare the way for the next succeeding series of changes that the food must undergo before it is absorbed.

In the mouth, food is reduced to a soft pulp by the mechanical action of the teeth, the tongue and cheeks. At the same time, the food is mixed with the saliva, which acts upon the starch, converting it into sugar. This action begins in the mouth and continues for one or two hours in the stomach after the food is swallowed.

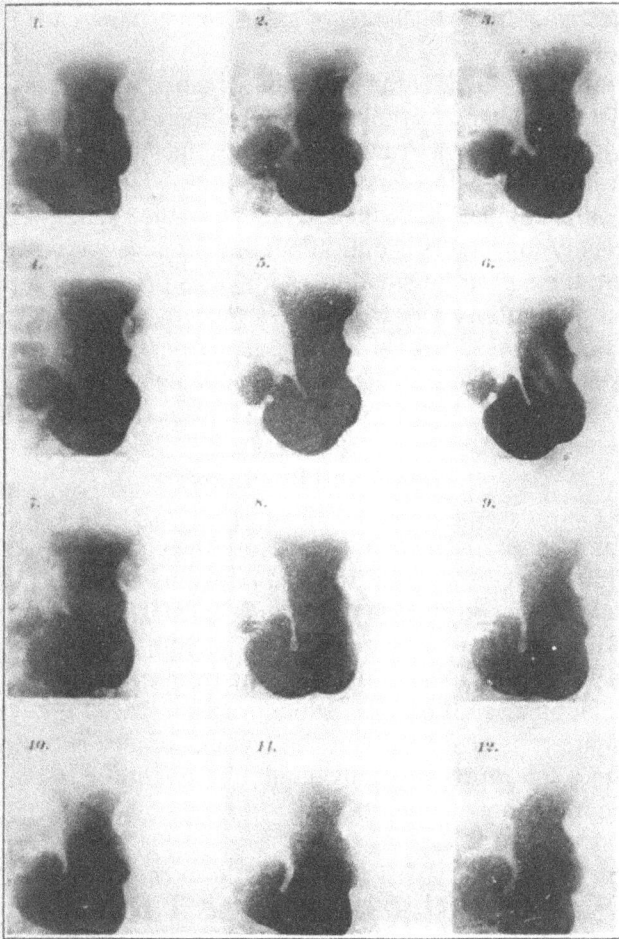

X-ray Motion Picture of the Stomach, showing Action of the Pylorus

In the stomach, the food is mixed with gastric juice, which, acting upon the food after it has been acted upon by the saliva, reduces it to a semi-fluid state. The mixing of the gastric juice with the food is accomplished by contraction waves, which pass along the stomach at the rate of three to five waves per minute.

These contraction waves also serve to pass the digested food into the small intestine through the pylorus in portions equal to about one tablespoonful.

The work of the stomach, like that of the mouth, is preliminary, having for its purpose the preparation of the food for further action by the digestive juices which it encounters in the small intestine.

In the small intestine, which is some twenty-two feet in length, is performed the greater part of the work of digestion, and practically the whole of the work of absorption. It is only in this part of the digestive apparatus that digestion is carried to the point of completion, by the action of the several quarts of digestive juices, consisting of gastric juice, pancreatic juice, intestinal juice, and the bile.

The small intestine absorbs the enormous quantity of five or six quarts of liquid daily. Of the solid matter taken at an ordinary meal, less than an ounce finds its way into the colon. Practically all the digestible and usable portion of the food is absorbed by the small intestine.

The total volume of material which passes from the small intestine into the colon each twenty-four hours is only about one pint.

It is evident, then, that the small intestine does practically all the work of digestion and absorption. The work performed by the stomach, while important, can be dispensed with. There are many persons living whose stomachs have been removed and who have good digestions, and enjoy good health.

The Food Residues

The small amount of matter that passes into the colon consists of indigestible food residues, excretory products and intestinal mucus. These substances are of no use to the body and may do much harm if retained because of the readiness with which they undergo putrefaction. It is the duty of the colon to receive these waste matters and dismiss them from the body.

During transit along the colon, a little more than half of the water content of the fecal matters is absorbed, but the amount of absorption which takes place from the colon represents only about one-twentieth of the work of absorption done by the small intestine.

The Digestive Time Table

Now that the work of the several departments of the alimentary canal has been defined, we are better prepared to understand the rhythmical processes by which nature moves the foodstuffs along from one part to another until all the usable material has been absorbed, and then disposes of the unusable residue.

Rhythmic Activity

The work of the stomach is completed in three to five hours, at the end of which time it is found empty.

The work of the small intestine, which begins within a few minutes after food is taken into the stomach, when the first small portions of liquid material begin to pass out through the pylorus, is finished at the end of eight or nine hours from the beginning of the meal.

At the end of eight hours in a normal person, the indigestible and unusable remnants of the food are found in the first part of the colon. Tests made by means of carmine, swallowed in a capsule, show that in normal persons, discharge of the unusable residues of the meal begins seven to ten hours after the meal is taken and may be completed in twelve to fourteen hours.

Rate of Movement

If the food can pass from the mouth to the colon, a distance of nearly twenty-five feet in eight hours, in the meantime undergoing the various complicated processes of gastric and intestinal digestion, there certainly seems to be no good reason why the food residue should not complete the transit of the colon, a distance only one-fifth as great, in one-half the time, or four hours, especially since the work done by the colon is almost exclusively mechanical, the work of digestion and absorption having been completed in the small intestine.

There seems to be no reason why the unusable remnants of the food should remain for many hours, even days, in the colon, undergoing putrefactive changes and contributing in no way whatever to the welfare of the body, but, on the contrary, serving as a tremendous vital handicap and a cause of multitudinous miseries, maladies, and degenerations.

Those who maintain that the normal time required for a meal to make the transit of the alimentary canal is forty-eight hours or more, should explain why it is necessary that the unusable remnants of a meal, the usable portion of which has been digested and absorbed in eight hours, should lie about rotting, putrefying and festering in the colon for forty hours or more, or five times the length of time required for digestion and absorption.

This long delay affords an opportunity for the development of putrefactive poisons, which not only Metchnikoff, but many other investigators, have shown to be the prime factors in the development of chronic disease and premature senility.

Nature's Plan

The writer has gathered from various sources a considerable amount of evidence that indicates that under normal conditions, a normal man, living upon a normal diet, which will include a sufficient amount of cellulose to furnish the normal stimulus to the muscular walls of the intestine, will experience an evacuation of alimentary wastes at least three times a day, and, in many cases, four times.

Three bowel movements a day, indeed, is the prevailing habit among primitive people and the higher apes. The chimpanzee and the orang-utan move their bowels four to six times daily.

15

This statement is made on information obtained by the writer direct from the keeper in charge of the London Zoo, to which several visits were made for the express purpose of inquiring into this matter and from others well acquainted with the habits of the big apes.

Doctor Hornaday, superintendent of the Bronx Park, informed the writer that the big monkeys of the Bronx zoological collection move their bowels three times daily.

When the intestine is empty, it is entirely quiet. When food is introduced into the stomach, contractile movements at once begin. These so-called peristaltic movements are not confined to the stomach, but simultaneously with the beginning of contractile waves in the stomach similar waves appear all along the intestinal tract, from stomach to colon.

Food Excites Peristalsis

Food is the natural laxative and the activity set up in the stomach by the taking of food, is communicated to the entire intestinal tract.

The result is that the intestinal activity set up by the taking of food into the stomach, not only serves to pass digesting food out of the stomach into the intestine but at the same time serves to move forward collections of food or food residues at various points in the alimentary canal.

When, for example, a mid-day meal is taken, a portion of the breakfast is still in the small intestine. The effect of peristaltic activity set up by the taking of the mid-day meal is to cause the small intestine to rapidly empty itself into the colon.

During the activity excited by luncheon or dinner, the residues of the breakfast, which have reached the colon, are gradually pushed farther along until at the end of eight or ten hours they reach the lower part of the colon.

When the morning meal is taken, a new series of vigorous peristaltic waves is set in motion. These not only push the unusable remnants of the last meal forward into the colon, but at the same time carry the residues of the breakfast to the lower part of the colon and thus create a desire for evacuation. This discharge of the unusable remnants of the breakfast should normally take place between dinner and supper or supper and bedtime.

That this rarely occurs is doubtless the result of too little roughage and neglect to attend promptly to the call of nature.

During the night, the residues of the last two meals of the day gradually work their way farther down and in the morning the intestinal activity naturally set up by the movements of the body on rising, should result in the discharge before breakfast of the residues of the mid-day meal of the day before. In the same way the vigorous peristaltic activity awakened by the taking of breakfast should result in the dismissal of the residues of the evening meal of the previous day.

In other words, the peristaltic wave set up by each meal should cause the advancement of the preceding meal from the small intestine into the colon, and, shortly afterward, the discharge of the unused remnants of the next to the last meal.

This is the normal intestinal rhythm and the nearer it can be approximated in actual experience, the better.

The writer is convinced that the highest degree of health, comfort, efficiency and longevity, can only be obtained by maintaining such a degree of intestinal activity as will prevent the accumulation in the colon of putrefying food residues and other poisonous wastes; for these putrefying materials contaminate the blood, and, by unnecessary and excessive work, wear out the liver, kidneys and other poison-destroying organs; damage the blood vessels by constant contact with a poison-laden blood current; and intoxicate and irritate, and ultimately render prematurely infirm and senile the body cells.

Normal Itinerary of a Meal Passing Through the Alimentary Subway

TIME TABLE

ARRIVAL	GATE	STATION	DEPARTURE
8:00 A.M.	No. 1. Food Administrator	Mouth	8:30 A.M.
	No. 2. Inspector		
	No. 3. Food and Water		
8:30 A.M.	No. 4. Stomach	Stomach	12:00 Noon
	No. 5. Bowel—Pylorus		
12:00 Noon	No. 6. Ileo. Sphincter	Small Intestine	4:00 P.M.
4:00 P.M.	No. 7. Colon–Ileo. Valve	Cecum	6:00 P.M.
6:00 P.M.	No. 8. Reversing Gate	Transverse Colon	8:00 P.M.
8:00 P.M.	No. 9. Ejector	Pelvic Colon	10:00 P.M.
	No. 10. Exit	Rectum	10:00 P.M.

SPECIAL NOTICES

Train Late: Held at Stomach Station for 2 hrs. Bowel Gate (No. 5) refused to open.

Losing Time: Wreck at Colon Gate (No. 7). Ileocecal valve refuses to close, track obstructed with rubbish. 8 hours late.

Losing Time: Collision with heavy train backing up. 10 hours late.

Losing Time: Obstruction on the track. Ejector Gate (No. 9) refuses to open. 20 hours late.

Losing Time: Serious obstruction. Track buried with rubbish. 35 hours late.

Train arrives at last, after clearing track with dynamite (castor oil), forty hours late.

(This is the usual program when the bowels move only once a day or occasionally.)

The Ten Gates

The study of the food gates is a new and highly interesting chapter in physiology which has been brought to light by the remarkable discoveries made by means of that magical revealer of secrets, the X-ray,

The movement of the food along the alimentary tube is not at a regular rate. Numerous pauses occur. The arrangement is similar to that of a well organized factory, in which a piece of mechanism, such as a watch for example, is passed from one to another of a long line of experts, each of whom does a particular part of the work, adding a wheel or a pinion, or some other necessary part, then passing the device along to the next workman, who advances the work another step towards completion.

The pauses essential for these special processes are secured by means of what may be called "gates," by which the progress of each morsel of food is temporarily checked while some special work, as of digestion, absorption, or selection, is being accomplished.

We are now somewhat acquainted with the food tube and its work, which consists essentially in passing the food along from one laboratory to another, finally gathering up the wastes and unusable residues and rejecting them from the body.

Let us now trace the progress of a test breakfast along the food tube and observe the ingenious devices by means of which the several processes are coordinated and the procession of body building and energy-feeding material maintained.

Many of the most serious disorders of digestion, recent physiological research has shown, are the result of disturbances which occur at the food gates, so that it is a matter of very great practical interest to discover the relation of these gates to healthy digestion, and to associate the various disturbances which occur in conditions of disease each with its particular gate.

The gates are ten in number. Their location and relation will be readily understood after a glance at the accompanying diagram.

The names of the several gates are as follows:

1. Entrance or Food Dictator's gate, the mouth.
2. Food Inspector's gate, the soft palate.
3. Food and Water gate.
4. Stomach gate.
5. The Bowel gate, Pylorus.
6. Control gate, ileocecal sphincter.
7. Colon gate, ileocecal valve.
8. Reversing gate, middle of transverse colon.
9. Discharging or ejector gate, pelvic colon.
10. Exit gate, anus.

Food Gate No. 1

The Entrance Gate — The Mouth

One purpose of the entrance gate is to guard the food tube and to keep out of it all harmful substances, rejecting of course, all things known to be poisonous, such as alcohol and tobacco, as well as tea and coffee and all other habit-forming drugs.

Just beneath the skin of the lips there is found a muscle entirely surrounding the mouth. This muscle is brought into strong action in whistling or puckering the lips. It normally acts with just sufficient force to keep the lips in contact when they are not open for the purpose of eating, drinking, or speaking. This is very necessary for maintaining a healthy condition of the mouth. When, for instance, the lower jaw drops down during sleep and the lips are parted, the air is drawn in through the mouth. The result may be serious injury to the throat through the excessive drying of the mucous membrane at the back of the throat, and still greater injury probably results from the infection which occurs as the result of the deposit of numerous germs on the surface of the tongue and pharynx.

The nose, which is the natural channel for the air in breathing, is provided with means for filtering and moistening air that is lacking in the mouth. In mouth breathing, numerous bacteria and microbic forms found in the air are deposited upon the tongue, soft palate, and the tonsils, and grow rapidly and produce overnight a thick foul coat upon the tongue, a disagreeable, unpleasant tasting slime which covers the teeth and all parts of the mouth.

On examination under a microscope this slime from the coating of the tongue shows bacteria in enormous numbers. Some of these are capable of living in the stomach when swallowed, as sometimes occurs during sleep, so infection may extend to the stomach and thence to the small intestine and the colon. These germs modern investigators have shown to be the cause of a large share of the maladies which afflict human beings in the civilized state, and are the cause of old age, as shown by Metchnikoff. In the Arctic region, where the air is free from germs, the intestines of animals are found to contain no bacteria.

The character of the material which passes along the food tube depends absolutely and wholly upon the action of the entrance gate in accepting or rejecting the various materials offered. The mouth is aided in its decisions by the sense of smell, by the memory of previous taste experiences and sometimes by common sense and reason. More often, the mouth lets in whatever is offered, or whatever a perverted appetite may call for.

Civilized people everywhere have cultivated many artificial and harmful appetites which call for the passage through the entrance gate of a multitude of substances which were never designed by nature to be eaten by human beings, as shown by the fact that they are not eaten by other animals belonging to the same biologic class with ourselves, that is the higher apes.

All horses adhere absolutely to a common bill of fare, that which has nourished their ancestors ever since horses appeared in the animal world.

Man is a primate, a member of a rather small family of animals which possess among other striking and peculiar characteristics, a pair of hands instead of feet attached to their anterior limbs. Nothing could be more evident than that man should adhere to the same dietary as his near relatives, the big apes, viz., fruits, nuts, tender green shoots, grains and succulent roots, adding milk and eggs.

Food Gate No. 2

The Inspector's Gate — The Soft Palate and Nerves of Taste

At the back of the mouth the palate and fauces combine to close the passage between the mouth and the pharynx, a small cavity in the upper part of the alimentary canal. This gate performs three important functions.

1. It insures thorough mastication of the food. The soft palate possesses peculiar sensibility to contact with solid objects. When such an object comes in contact with the uvula a reflex action is at once produced, as the result of which the base of the tongue is drawn up and the object thrown forward into the mouth. Strong stimulation of the fauces produces coughing and gagging, by which solid materials may be projected forward with so much force as to be ejected from the mouth. This is the reason why it is difficult to swallow a pill, for which, indeed, some practice is necessary in the case of many persons.

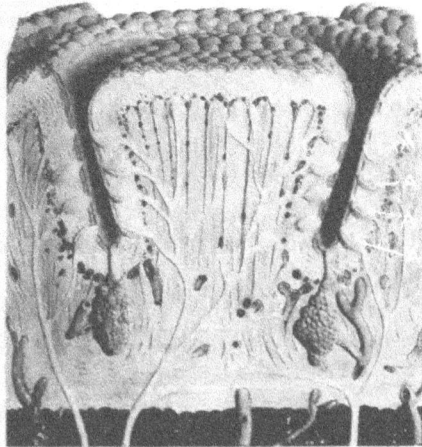

Cross-section of Papilla from back of Tongue showing Taste Buds at A.

Now below the mouth the alimentary canal provides no means for the mechanical reduction of the food. Certain birds are provided with a mill lower down — the gizzard, — and in some lower species of animals more complicated mechanisms are provided for grinding the food. Such animals naturally swallow their food entire, but in human beings, as well as in the horse and most other mammals, the mill is located in the mouth, and it is the duty of the soft palate to see that the food is completely ground and reduced to a semiliquid state before it is permitted to proceed further along the digestive tract. Thorough mastication is necessary in order that the saliva and the juices of the stomach and intestine may be readily brought into contact with every particle of food, so that each may do its work upon the individual food elements promptly and completely.

That the jaws were intended for powerful action is shown by the extraordinary power which their muscles possess. The strength of the bite is seldom less than eighty pounds and sometimes reaches two hundred and fifty pounds.

2. The inspector's gate holds the food in the mouth long enough for the nerves of taste to exercise their functions. Pavlov, of Petrograd, discovered that the nerves of taste with which the food is brought in contact in the mouth, perform a most important function in relation to the digestion of food in the stomach. At the back of the tongue there is found an interesting arrangement by which the nerves of taste are brought in direct contact with dissolved particles of food. It is evident, however, that the food must be finely divided in order that such contact may be made. These extraordinarily sensitive taste nerves detect the special properties of food, and when stimulated, arouse the activity of the nerve-centers in the brain, so called "psychic centers," and send messages to the stomach, in response to which the gastric glands produce "appetite juice."

The amount of appetite juice depends upon the extent to which the gustatory nerves are stimulated, and this depends wholly upon the thoroughness with which the food is masticated, for the flavor of the food cannot be detected by the gustatory nerves unless the food has been dissolved. The sweetness of a lump of sugar, for instance, cannot be appreciated until the sugar has been brought into solution.

Nature has given to the various natural foods just the flavors required to stimulate the gustatory nerve sufficiently to cause the production of the proper quantity and quality of gastric juice required to digest the food. In other words, when the food is swallowed in masses, as one might swallow pills or capsules, the flavors are swallowed with it, and the gustatory nerve has no opportunity to inspect and become acquainted with the food; the stomach, accordingly, receives no intimation of what sort of food is coming, and is unprepared to receive it.

3. Still another function of the inspector's gate is to regulate the quality of food. Our food is a complicated substance. It consists of combinations in various proportions of proteins, fats, and carbohydrates, together with flavoring materials and various mineral salts, which, while essential, play a minor part in nutrition. The proportion of these food elements is constantly varying, even in foodstuffs similar in character; for example, wheat flour consists chiefly of gluten, protein, and starch (a carbohydrate), but no two flours con-

tain the same proportion of gluten and starch, and so every loaf of bread differs from every other loaf. Chemists can make an analysis by which the composition of every foodstuff or every particular particle of food may be exactly known, but such an analysis could not be made for every meal.

The body requires a more reliable guide than can be afforded by the chemical laboratory, or the most exact dietetic knowledge, and so we find that so long as an animal subsists upon those articles of food which are natural to it and normally adapted to its digestive organs and constitution, the gustatory nerves, cooperating with Food Gate No. 2, are able to meet the nutritive needs of the body in a manner incomparably better than could be done by the most astute dietitian.

When the food is swallowed in haste without thorough mastication, there is no opportunity for regulation. Regulation is, indeed, impossible. When, however, the food is masticated thoroughly so that the gustatory nerves have an opportunity to inspect every particle of food, then regulation will be most complete. One who uses his palate gate normally, eating natural food and chewing it so thoroughly that it may be completely tasted before it is swallowed, does not need to ascertain by means of scales or chemical analysis how much fat or protein or carbohydrates he is taking at a meal. He can depend with confidence upon the efficiency of automatic regulation through his gustatory nerves.

The inspector's gate should be given a chance to examine the foodstuffs and its mandates should be obeyed.

When the food has been properly chewed, that is, brought to a soft, liquid consistency, it slips by the food inspector's gate so easily that it appears to be swallowed automatically and without effort.

The nerves of the soft palate seem to possess extraordinary wisdom in relation to the needs of the body and not only observe the way in which the food has been chewed, but also its various dietetic properties, and in a marvelously efficient way cater to the real needs of the body. By this means the inspector gate becomes, to a very large degree, the regulator of the body's nutrition.

Food Gate No. 3

The Food and Water Gate

There are at the back of the throat two gates, one, the epiglottis or air gate, which controls the passage of air to the lungs and excludes water or solid substances; a second gate which closes the upper end of the esophagus or gullet and only opens for the passage of food and drink in swallowing, and excludes air from the stomach.

The food and water gate is formed by the pressure of the larynx against the gullet, compressing it against the spinal column. The gate is opened by the act of swallowing. This act is normally executed only when food or drink are brought in contact with the mucous membrane of the back of the throat. Foreign or obnoxious substances provoke gagging, coughing, or choking, by which the objectional matters are ejected. The food and water gate refuses to open to receive them unless forced to do so by a violent effort.

This gate thus affords important and intelligent protection against injury from foreign substances not intended by nature to be taken into the body. The protest of the gate is so strong that sometimes vomiting may be induced. Tickling the throat with the finger or a feather is a common means of provoking vomiting when it is desirable to empty the stomach.

On the other hand, the readiness with which wholesome foods and drinks are received is quite remarkable. A partial vacuum is maintained in the gullet just within the gate, by the elasticity of the lungs, so that the instant it is opened by the act of swallowing which lifts the larynx forward and upward and so removes the pressure on the gullet, the food is drawn in instantly by the suction, and with so much force that it is sometimes carried nearly to the lower end of the gullet. This remarkable arrangement accounts for the suddenness, often very surprizing, with which substances which reach the back of the throat are sometimes snatched away from voluntary control, and even when imperfectly masticated, so that more or less distress may be felt as the mass is slowly passed along the gullet to the stomach.

The act of breathing is always arrested during the swallowing of food or liquid, this being necessary not only for the protection of the lungs, but also to prevent the entrance of air into the stomach with the food, since the opening of the oesophageal gate permits the suction effect to operate through the oesophagus as well as through the larynx. If the breath is strongly drawn in at the same time the gate is opened by swallowing, air may be drawn into the oesophagus. After the gate is again closed, the air taken into the oesophagus is gradually forced into the stomach, into which it enters with a characteristic sound, which is usually audible at a distance of some feet.

Nervous persons suffering from disordered digestion often acquire the habit of pumping air into the stomach in this way, a symptom technically termed "aerophagy." Horses often acquire this habit and in farm parlance are called "cribbers," "wind suckers," or "stump suckers," for the reason that they forcibly seize some object with the teeth when swallowing air.

Air swallowing is somewhat akin to hiccough, but it is more subject to voluntary control than is hiccough. It is induced by a feeling of fullness in the stomach which is mistaken for an accumulation of gas, whereas it is an irritation often due to excessive acidity of the gastric secretions. Temporary relief is obtained by forcing air into the stomach, but soon the stomach becomes distended and then belching occurs, which confirms the idea that the trouble is due to "gas on the stomach," whereas there is usually no considerable amount of gas in the stomach until air has been swallowed.

The disposition to swallow air should be restrained.

When the unpleasant sensation is experienced, the mouth should be held widely open while ten deep breaths are taken. It is also well to drink a glassful of hot water. The symptom is often due to hyperacidity from excessive secretion of gastric acid, which should be relieved by the proper measures.

Food Gate No. 4

The Stomach Gate

At the lower end of the gullet is a circular muscle which surrounds the tube and tightly closes the gullet after food has passed through it into the stomach. When food coming down the gullet approaches the stomach gate, the muscle relaxes; that is, the gate opens to allow the food to pass into the stomach, then instantly closes.

This circular muscle sometimes becomes relaxed to such a degree that portions of food may be forced back into the oesophagus by movements of the stomach, and thus find their way back to the mouth. This usually happens when the contents of the stomach are too highly acid, because of the excessive secretion of hydrochloric acid by the gastric glands. In some persons the muscle appears to be weakened and relaxed through the habit of drinking large quantities of warm water, which produce nausea and regurgitation, or even by vomiting as the result of tickling the throat with the finger or a feather.

Eructations of gas from the stomach are usually due to the fact that the cardiac orifice, or upper stomach gate, is not sufficiently strong to resist the violent movements of the stomach induced by an excess of acid in the stomach and resulting too tight closure of the pylorus. When the stomach is in a state of inflammation, and ulceration exists in the upper part of the stomach, this gate becomes abnormally sensitive and pain is experienced after the swallowing of food or drink, due to the passage of the food over the irritated surfaces.

Food Gate No. 5

The Bowel Gate — the Pylorus

This is a most remarkable structure. It consists of a circular muscle which surrounds the food tube at the point of junction between the stomach and the small intestine. From the most ancient times some knowledge of the function of the pylorus has existed, hence its Greek name, which translated into English is simply gate keeper.

This, of all the gateways through which the food passes, has been the subject of the greatest amount of study, but it is only within recent years that the function of the pylorus has been properly understood.

The pylorus inspects the digesting food stuffs, opening at proper intervals to allow the passage into the bowel of such portions of the food as have been prepared by the stomach for the more complete digestion in the small intestine.

A very interesting point about this gate is the manner of its closing or control. When the stomach is empty, the gate remains open. This is also true in cases in which the stomach has through disease lost the power of making gastric juice, so-called cases of *achylia.*

Water or other liquids with a temperature near that of the body when taken into the stomach quickly flow out through the pylorus into the intestine. The normal position of the stomach is known to be perpendicular, obviously to facilitate the downward movement of the liquid contents.

When, however, food is taken into the stomach, even while it is still undergoing mastication in the mouth, the acid gastric juice entering the duodenum causes the pylorus to contract. This closure of the lower food gate is necessary to cause the retention of the food in the stomach until it has been acted upon by the saliva and gastric juice, and thus prepared for the digestive processes which later on take place along the alimentary canal at certain intervals.

In normal persons, when the acid contents of the stomach begin to pass out into the small intestine, a reflex action occurs which closes the pylorus. The contact of the acid with the mucous membranes causes contraction and closure of the pylorus which continues until the gastric acid has been neutralized by the alkaline bile and pancreatic juice, then the pylorus relaxes and lets out into the intestine another small quantity of gastric contents.

By this wonderful arrangement the food which has undergone digestion in the stomach is doled out into the intestine in very small portions, a provision entirely in harmony with the now known fact that this function is chiefly preparatory, the complete and finished work of digestion being accomplished only in the intestine.

The stomach was formerly supposed to be the chief organ of digestion. It is now known that this idea was erroneous. The stomach is a highly useful organ, but not essential. In many cases practically the whole stomach has been removed in cases of cancer involving a large part of the organ, and a considerable number of persons have lived in this condition for years in comfortable health.

Numerous digestive disorders may be traced to the pyloric gate, through which all foodstuffs must pass before they can take part in the nutrition of the body. When the contents of the stomach become excessively acid, the pylorus contracts so forcibly that the digested portions of the food are not passed on, but are retained in the stomach. This is a difficulty which serves to aggravate itself. A vicious circle is formed. The excessive acidity of the gastric contents causes too long a retention of the foodstuffs in the stomach, and the long delay of food in the stomach irritates the gastric glands, causing an abnormal secretion of acid. Thus, the difficulty once begun tends to become worse. The stomach muscles contract with increased vigor as the acidity increases, and not infrequently the movements become so violent that a portion of the acid contents of the stomach is forced upward through the esophagus into the mouth, giving rise to eructations of gas, and even liquid or solid food materials, accompanied by a burning pain. Here we have the explanation of so-called "heartburn," which has been erroneously attributed to fermentation in the stomach — a rare condition.

There are thus many causes which may disturb the passage of food through the pyloric gate, all of which give rise to serious disturbances of the digestive processes. Many chronic dyspeptics suffer from some of these conditions, which, however, in most cases cannot be remedied by the use of drugs or internal remedies of any sort, since the obstruction is due to spasm of the pylorus, the result of excessive acid secretion by the stomach. Regulation of the diet and other proper modes of treatment will almost certainly give relief. In cases in which the stomach is prolapsed, the restoration of the stomach to its normal place, and the use of a suitable bandage will often secure very great improvement. It is not possible to say in many cases just which one of various causes exists, without a thorough examination of the stomach by means of a test meal and careful chemical examination of gastric contents, together with an X-ray bismuth meal examination, by means of which the stomach may be clearly outlined and its movements, together with its location and the action of the pylorus, clearly seen.

X-ray examinations have clearly established the fact that in a great number of cases, distress and other symptoms attributed to the stomach are due to causes outside of the stomach altogether. For example, gall stones, inflammation of the gallbladder, ulcer of the duodenum, and inflammation of the pancreas, and even infection of the appendix and colitis, often give rise to gastric pain and other disturbances of the stomach. These extrinsic disorders constitute possibly one-half of all gastric cases. These cases are, in fact, so common, it may be regarded as a very wise and helpful procedure to submit every case of chronic gastric disease to a critical X-ray examination by the aid of the "barium meal," in addition to the ordinary gastric test meal.

One of the functions of the acid gastric juice is to cause closure of the pylorus and regulation of the action of this remarkable structure in "spooning" the food from the stomach into the intestine. In cases in which the gastric glands have degenerated so that no hydrochloric acid is produced, the pylorus remains open. In cancer of the stomach and in certain cases of ulceration of the stomach, the disease may be located in such a position as to prevent the normal closure of the pylorus. Similar conditions are sometimes produced by adhesions of the pylorus to the liver or gall bladder, a result of inflammation of the gall ducts or gall bladder.

A relaxed condition of the pylorus gate that prevents its proper closure may be a cause of serious disturbance. When this condition is present, bile frequently flows back into the stomach, especially when the stomach is prolapsed. The food passes out of the stomach so quickly that the work of the stomach upon the food is not properly performed, and in consequence digestion in the intestines is deranged. In such cases a movement of the bowels sometimes occurs within a half hour after eating, discharging food of the last meal.

Food Gate No. 6

The Food Control Gate — The Ileocecal Sphincter

A muscular ring much like the pylorus surrounds the lower end of the small intestine. This structure, the ileocecal sphincter, performs very much the same function as the pylorus. The pylorus holds the food in the stomach until gastric digestion is completed and the food prepared for intestinal digestion. The ileocecal sphincter holds the food in the small intestine until the work of digestion is completed and the digested food stuffs absorbed. The matters passed into the colon by the sphincter are the undigested and unused or unusable food remnants and wastes, along with a considerable amount of water (90%) and very small amounts of digested or partly digested foodstuffs, with mucus and certain excretory substances eliminated by the liver in the bile, and by the intestinal mucous membrane.

If this gate did not exist, the liquid food stuffs which leave the stomach would pass rapidly through the whole food tube and would be discharged before opportunity had been given for absorption.

The intelligent and efficient regulation of the flow of waste matters into the colon, is highly essential for the proper nutrition of the body and render this little muscle wholly deserving of the very honorable title of food controller or control gate.

Food Gate No. 7

The Colon Gate or the Ileocecal Valve.

This is a very simple and at the same time an exceedingly important and interesting structure. The ileocecal valve was discovered and described by anatomists more than 300 years ago (1579 A.D.). The discoverers recognized at once the fact that this curious structure was designed to act as a check valve, that is, a gate opening in but one direction.

Modern anatomical studies have shown that all animals possessed of a backbone, that is, all vertebrate animals, are furnished with an ileocecal valve.

This gate is necessary for two highly important reasons. First, to maintain a definite and steady forward movement of the intestinal contents; and second, to prevent the return into the small intestine of waste and excretory matters after they have been rejected by the small intestine and pushed into the colon to be cast out of the body as refuse.

The importance of this wise provision of nature grows out of the fact that the waste matters passed into the colon very readily take on putrefactive processes and thus become highly offensive and poisonous.

The colon is provided with means of defense against these poisons and is thus prepared to serve the purpose of a sewer for the body without serious injury either to itself or the body. But this is not true of the small intestine with its highly delicate mucous membrane and exceedingly active absorbing structures. The result, in fact, when foul, putrefying fecal matters enter the small intestine from the colon, is not much different from what might be expected if feces were mixed with the food and taken in by the mouth. The small intestine not only rapidly absorbs the poisonous matters but becomes infected by the virulent bacteria which are present.

The infection travels upward and may reach the gall bladder, causing inflammation and gall-stones or disease of the pancreas and may cause ulcer of the stomach or duodenum. More common results of the entrance of fecal matters into the small intestine are attacks of headache, skin eruptions, depression, nervous exhaustion, asthmatic attacks, so-called "bilious" attacks, a coated tongue and bad breath and probably chronic disease of the blood vessels, heart, kidneys and other vital organs.

All these and other troubles follow when the colon gate fails to shut through becoming incompetent, a condition which often results from chronic constipation, as will be shown later on.

The action of the colon gate is very simple. It is in fact quite mechanical in its action. The valve consists of two membranous lips which project into the colon from the borders of the junction of the small intestine with the colon. When matters pass from the small intestine into the colon, the lips separate, offering no resistance to the forward movement. But when the slightest back pressure occurs with a movement of matters toward the small intestine, the lips fall together and form an impassable barrier. In other words, the colon gate is highly efficient as a check valve.

This is true, however, only when the valve is intact. It is apparently more liable to injury and derangement than any other of the several gates which regulate the movement of material along the food tube. When waste matters are allowed to accumulate in the lower half of the colon, which occurs in all cases of constipation, the right half of the colon is over-filled with feces and over-distended with gases, and the caecum in time becomes dilated and pouched and the colon gate is so damaged that it does not close.

The foul fecal matters in the colon pass back into the small intestine and all the serious consequences which have been traced to autointoxication or intestinal toxemia are the natural consequence.

It is quite possible that more human suffering, physical and mental, has resulted from the breaking down of the colon gate than from any other common injury.

The chief cause of injury to the colon gate is constipation, a disease which is practically universal among civilized human beings, and equally universal among house dogs. "Housebroken" dogs are usually constipated, and for the same reason as their house-broken masters, viz., voluntary interference with the normal, rhythmical and automatic action of the food tube by which its contents are moved along and unusable residues rejected. More will be said on this phase of the subject later.

By appropriate diet and treatment, the evil effects of incompetency of the ileocecal valve may be very largely overcome and a radical cure may be effected by means of a simple and safe but somewhat delicate operation.

Food Gate No. 8

The Reversing Gate

Near the middle of the transverse colon there is located a remarkable structure which originates rhythmical movements in the intestine just as a similar nerve structure near the heart produces the regular beating of the heart.

A most remarkable characteristic of the movements starting at the middle of the transverse colon is the fact that they extend in both directions. That is, a series of contraction waves moves forward toward the exit while another series moves at the same time in the opposite direction, toward the caecum. These latter, known as antiperistaltic waves, hold the liquid wastes in the caecum until a large part of the water which they contain has been absorbed. This reduces the volume of the feces and secures periodical emptying of the colon instead of continuous or very frequent discharge of the thin liquid matters which enter the colon from the small intestine.

At intervals the antiperistaltic waves cease and the contents of the caecum and ascending colon are pushed forward by strong contractions of the caecum. That portion which reaches a point far enough beyond the center of the transverse colon to be caught in the outgoing current is carried on to the exit; but a considerable portion does not reach this point and is swept back into the caecum by the antiperistaltic waves.

The action of the antiperistaltic waves brings pressure against the colon gate, the ileocecal valve. A normal valve easily resists the pressure and prevents the antiperistaltic waves from forcing fecal matters back into the small intestine. But when the valve has been broken down and rendered incompetent by chronic constipation, nothing hinders the reflux into the small intestine produced by the antiperistaltic contractions which are almost constantly active in the right half of the colon, especially during and for some time after a meal.

When fecal matters accumulate in the lower half of the colon, the antiperistaltic action is much increased. This is also true in case of colitis and after the use of laxative or cathartic drugs.

Food Gate No. 9

The Discharging or Ejector Gate — The Pelvic Colon

Here is another most interesting gate which is charged with a highly important function, the periodical discharge of the food residues and other wastes.

The Pelvic Colon is the loop of the large intestine which joins the rectum. It is not closely attached to the abdominal wall as are the descending and the iliac colon, but has a long mesentery (the membrane by which it is attached to the back of the abdominal cavity). This arrangement permits considerable freedom of movement. The bowel falls down collapsed after a bowel movement, then gradually rises as it fills and when sufficiently distended pushes some of its contents into the rectum and so evokes the act of defecation.

In this way the pelvic colon operates a periodical discharging process, an automatic "dumping" or ejection of the body wastes, and so may be very properly termed the discharging or ejector gate. As we shall see later, this important gate is sometimes crippled so that it does not operate efficiently. When fallen down after defecation, it becomes caught and may even become adherent so that it cannot rise and thus the discharging apparatus of the colon is thrown out of commission and a very obstinate form of constipation is the result. Fortunately the difficulty may be radically remedied by an appropriate surgical operation. In most cases palliative measures give practical relief.

Food Gate No. 10

The Exit Gate — the Anus

The anal sphincter is controlled by nerve centers which maintain it in a state of constant contraction except during bowel movement. When an expulsion wave travels down the pelvic colon, the center controlling the anal sphincter causes it to relax so that it offers no resistance to the discharge of the bowel contents.

The presence of hemorrhoids, ulcer, fissure, catarrh of the rectum, and other causes may so irritate the anal muscle that it will contract with too great vigor, or even spasm may be produced, and thus a "tight sphincter" may become a cause of constipation by closing the exit gate so tightly that it will not open under the stimulus of the normal reflex. It is possible that ovarian, bladder, prostatic and other pelvic disorders may cause anal contraction and so oppose normal bowel movement.

The "House-Broken" Colon

We are all born wild.

Civilization is a process of taming and is often so overdone as to become destructive.

No other animal except the house-dog suffers from constipation as does man; and the dog suffers from colon troubles for the same reason the man does, namely, because he is "house-broken."

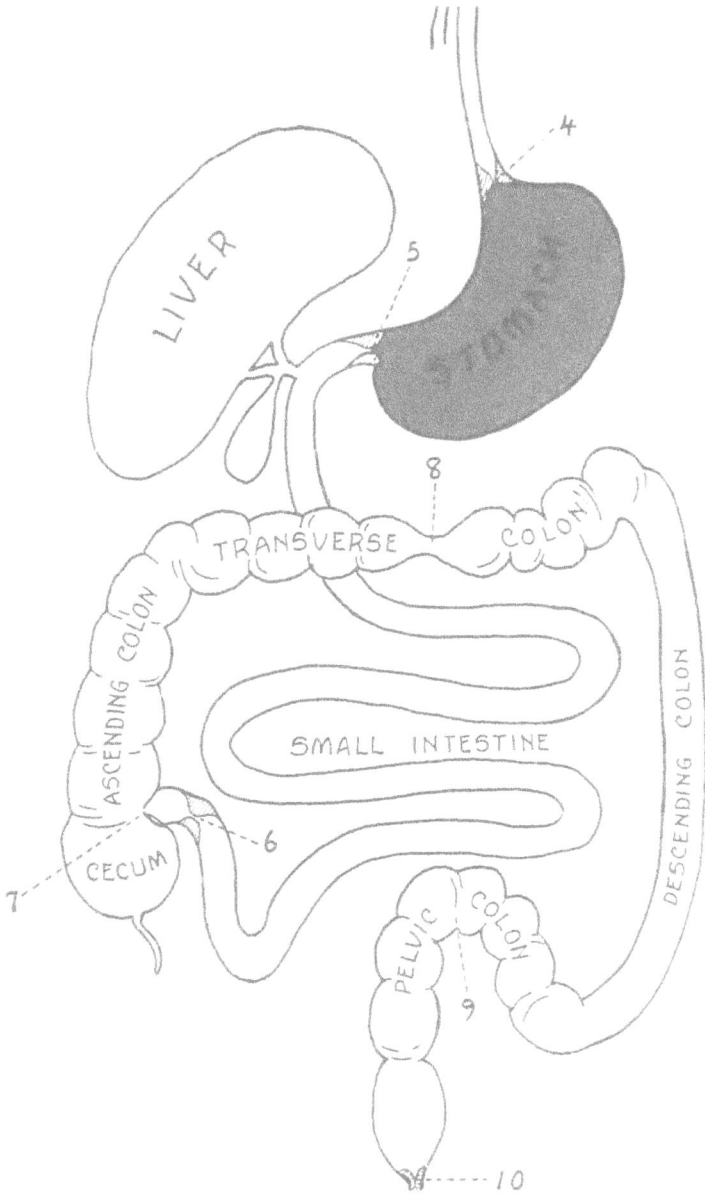

8:00 - 9:00 A. M. Breakfast (shaded) just Eaten.

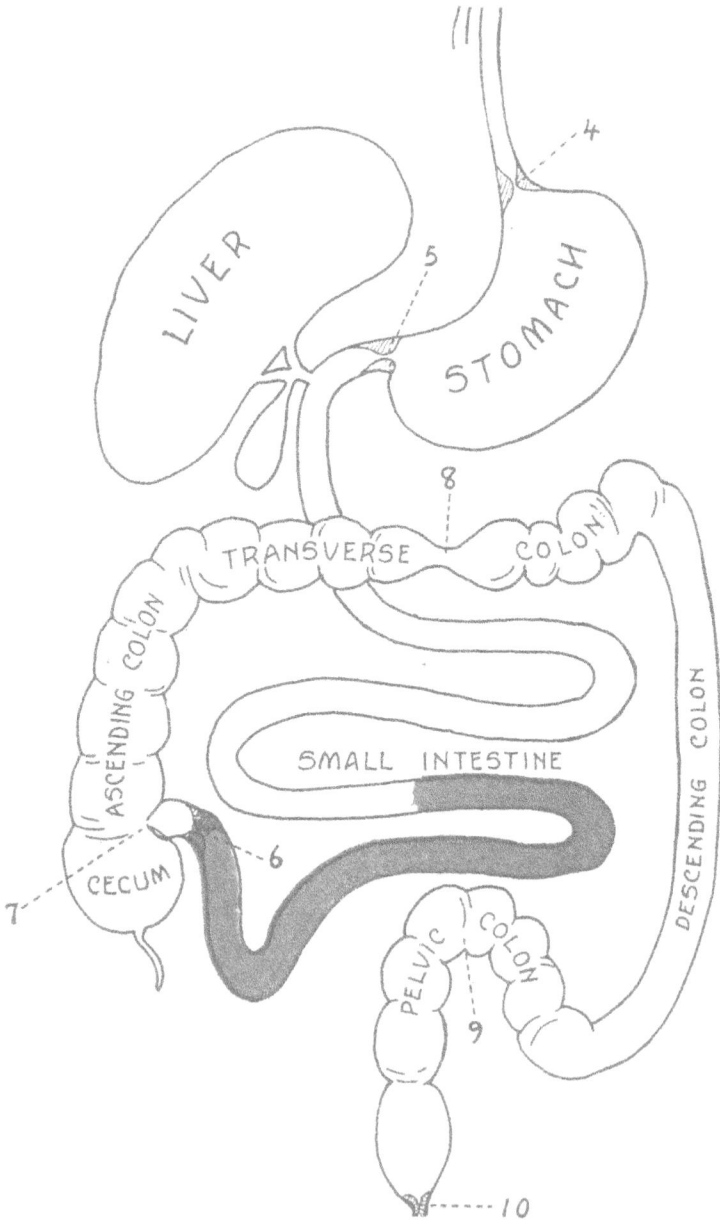

12:00 Noon

Breakfast (shaded), four hours after eating, has reached lower end of small intestine and ileocecal sphincter. Digestion and absorption of food are completed, and the unusable residue is ready to be passed into the colon.

The wild man and the wild dog, as well as man's nearest relatives, the big apes, of the African jungles, know nothing of the miseries of constipation, colon stasis, or constipation, a product of civilization. It is the result of perverted habits, neglect, and pernicious training and education.

The civilized colon is a poor cripple, maimed, misshapen, overstretched in parts, contracted in other parts, prolapsed, adherent, "kinked," infected, paralyzed, inefficient, incompetent. It is the worst abused and the most variously damaged of any organ of the body.

Before the advent of the X-ray, no one had more than a suspicion of the sad condition of the poor colon. It was known to be generally inefficient, but this was charged to inertia, a sort of constitutional laziness rather than to definite disease or structural damage.

But the X-ray, that marvelous revealer of secrets, has given us a look inside and has revealed a state of depravity in the colon never dreamed of. In the light of modern X-ray revelations, the colon appears to have more different and serious things the matter with it than any other bodily organ.

Now that the X-ray has made clear to us the physiology of the colon and has shown us the numerous deformities and incompetences of the average civilized colon, thanks to the exhaustive studies of Cannon, Hirsch, Case, and other roentgenologists, we have come to know that constipation is not a simple disease but is instead, a highly complex condition or rather a symptom which may result from a very considerable number of clearly defined diseased conditions and combinations of conditions.

Normal Bowel Action

Evacuation of the bowels is the result of two forces acting upon the bowel contents, viz.:

(1) Compression of the bowels by the abdominal walls and the diaphragm.

(2) Contraction of the bowel itself.

In natural bowel movement the squatting position is assumed. In this position the pressure of the thighs upon the abdomen compresses the bowel. At the same time the diaphragm is forced downward by a deep, prolonged breath and the abdominal muscles are voluntarily contracted.

These are the preliminary movements which precede actual evacuation. They often fail, and usually do in cases of marked constipation. Under normal conditions, however, evacuation quickly follows the preliminary efforts through actions set up by the defecating center. When the voluntary efforts result in forcing fecal matter from the pelvic colon into the rectum, a new series of movements begin. The presence of feces in the rectum sets up a reflex nerve action through the defecating center by which the abdominal muscles are made to contract with greater force, the colon itself contracts either in part or in its entirety, the anus relaxes, and finally the levator ani, a muscle attached to the rectal walls, contracts in such a manner as to insure complete emptying of the rectum.

This normal bowel movement should leave the rectum and at least the left half of the colon, completely empty. And this complete emptying should take place after every meal for the reason that after each meal the unused residues of the preceding meal but one, are normally deposited in the pelvic colon ready to be dismissed from the body. That is, the discharge gate or dumping device of the colon is loaded and ought to be "dumped." There is no possible benefit to be derived from retaining the excretory and unusable residues, and if retained they do harm through the absorption of putrefaction poisons which are thus produced. Besides, these wastes are the best sort of soil for the growth of highly active pathological or disease-producing species of germs, streptococci and other pus forming germs which attach themselves to the wall of the bowel and set up that very serious and very common disease, colitis.

Hindrances to Normal Bowel Action

Now that we know how the bowels should move, let us see what causes interfere with normal bowel action, that is, let us seek an answer to the question, Why is the civilized man unable to evacuate his bowels three or four times daily or after each meal, as does the savage or the semi-civilized man and our near relatives in the family of primates, the orang and the chimpanzee?

There are many causes, chief of which, perhaps, are the following, referred to in the order in which they operate rather than their relative importance:

1. *The Sitting Posture:* The savage evacuates in a crouching or squatting position. Semi-civilized people and the peasantry of civilized nations do the same. In the homes of the poor classes and in country inns and even in the small city hotels of France and Italy, as well as countries farther East, the toilet conveniences consist simply of a hole in the floor and a large pipe connecting it with a receptacle below.

The toilet seat which civilization has provided as more elegant and convenient, has proved to be a prolific cause of constipation with all its miseries and inconveniences through loss of the thigh pressure against the abdomen, one of the important initial efforts in bowel movement.

It is not necessary to return to the primitive form of toilet convenience, but toilet seats should be low and should have a backward slope. An efficient remedy for the defects of the ordinary closet seat is found in placing before the seat a stool about eight inches high to support the feet.

2. *Weak Abdominal Muscles:* A sedentary life, general lack of muscular development, and especially the "slumped" or "stooped" position in sitting and working, result in a weak and relaxed condition of the abdominal muscles so that they are not able to do their part in pushing forward the contents of the lower colon into the rectum and thus starting the automatic process by which the colon itself contracts and empties itself. This condition is practically universal among civilized women because of their mode of dress and defi-

cient muscular activity. Professional men, clerks, students, bookkeepers and factory workers suffer from the same cause.

One very serious result of weakness of the abdominal muscles is the prolapse of the colon, stomach, liver and other heavy organs of the abdomen. While it is true, as shown in recent years, that these organs are able to do their work quite efficiently even though prolapsed, great mischief results from the fact that in falling they drag down with them the diaphragm, the great muscle which forms the floor of the chest and is the great air pump of the body. In doing its work the diaphragm rises and falls. The broader its swing the greater the amount of air moved.

When held down by prolapsed viscera, the diaphragm cannot rise high into the chest as it should and consequently the lungs cannot be well emptied.

On the other hand, not being able to rise properly, it has not room for downward movement, and so the low-standing diaphragm not only fails to fill the lungs but also fails to do its part in emptying the bowels. So persons with weak abdominal muscles easily get out of breath and are constipated.

Weak abdominal muscles may be made strong by such exercises as raising both legs while lying on the back, repeating the movement thirty or forty times morning and night. The chest must be held high so as to keep the abdominal muscles stretched to their full length and thus afford them an opportunity for action. This requires constant attention to posture when at work and the use of a chair which properly supports the hollow of the back and holds the chest up when the body is relaxed.

Deep breathing, wearing a spring abdominal supporter, exercises with the head low (inclined plane exercises) and the use of the weighted compress, are the means by which this cause of constipation may be combated.

Vigorous bodily exercises of all sorts, including walking, and especially hill climbing and such sports as golf, volley ball, lawn tennis, rowing and swimming, are excellent aids to bowel action. It should be remarked, however, that the excessive perspiration produced by vigorous exercise tends to cause constipation.

The importance of the above named faulty habits as causes of constipation will be appreciated only when it is remembered that in health the rectum is always empty. The pelvic loop which lies just above the rectum is the end of the colon reservoir. In normal defecation the fecal matters are pushed forward from the colon into the rectum by voluntary effort. When this fails, the feces remain in the colon and in time become hard and dry by the absorption of moisture. When this stage is reached the feces can not be pushed along my compression of the bowels and an enema or a laxative is required to empty the colon. If the retention and drying is less prolonged, the result is the so-called "well-formed stool," which is positive proof of constipation as it can only be produced by retention and drying of the colon contents. The "well-formed stool" has become almost a fetish with many persons, even some doctors. A western doctor actually advises his patients to resist a disposition to bowel movement in the evening, "to save it 'till morning" so as to secure a well-formed stool. Such notions are based upon ignorance. Nature's suggestion of the need of bowel movement should never be resisted or thwarted except in emergency and when unavoidable.

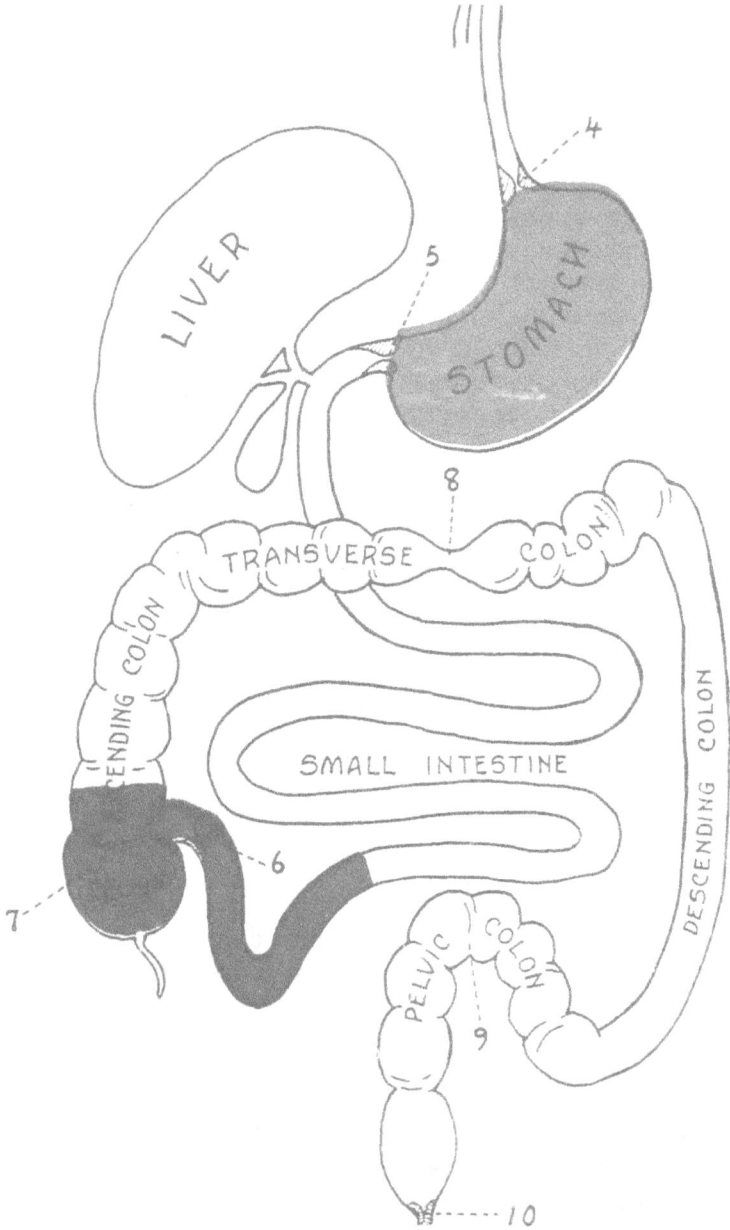

1:00 P. M.
Breakfast Residue (dark) is passing into the Colon. Dinner (shaded), just eaten, is in the Stomach.

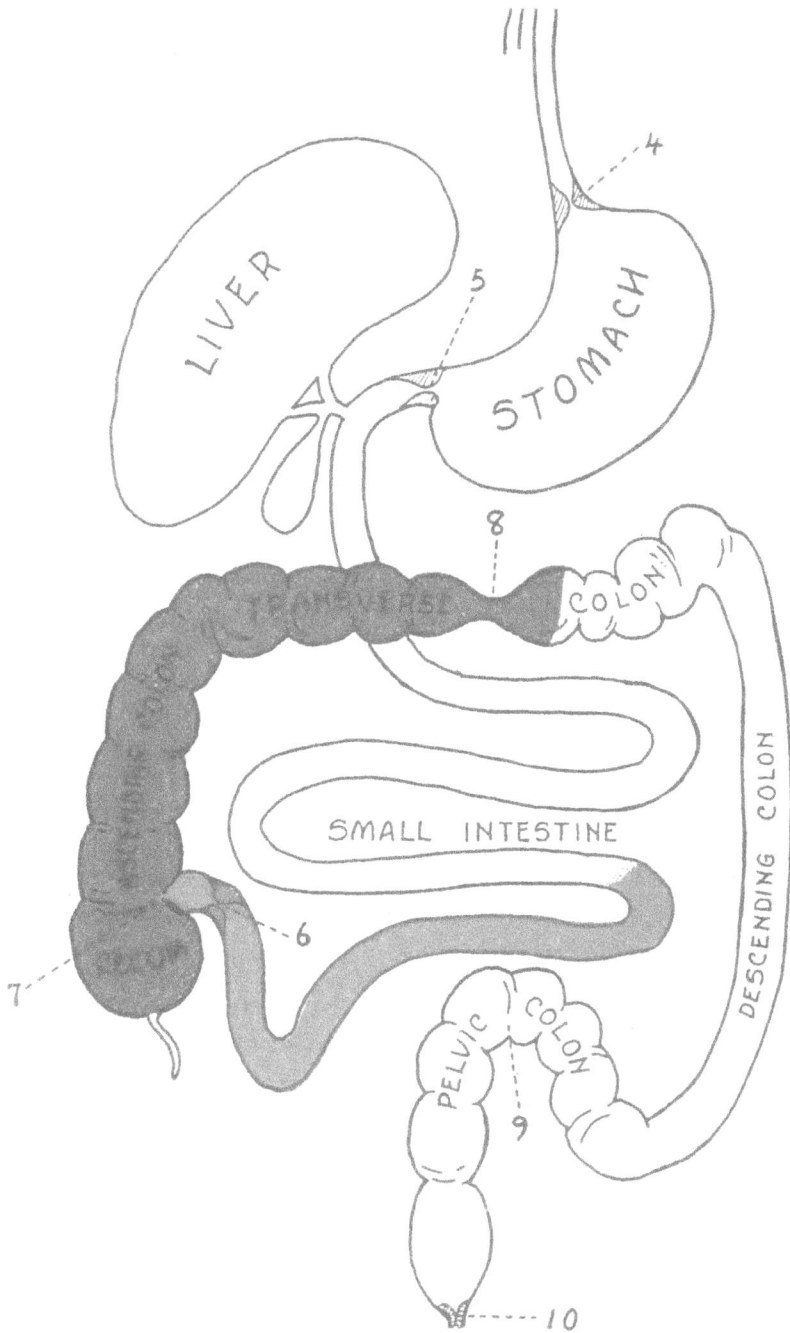

5:00 P. M.
Breakfast Residue (dark) all in Colon. Dinner Residue (shaded) Ready to enter Colon.

3. *A Concentrated Diet:* The human food tube is adapted to a rather coarse and bulky diet, less coarse and bulky than that of the herbivorous animals, such as the ox and the goat, but much more bulky than that of the dog, cat and other carnivora. This is shown by the long alimentary canal and capacious colon. The intestine of the sheep is thirty times its body length, that of the cat only three and a half times, and that of the shark merely the length of the body, simply a straight tube with a single short loop.

The human food tube is ten times the length of the body, and the colon is of large proportions. In animals the diet of which is very concentrated, the colon almost disappears.

Man is a primate, that is a relative of the chimpanzee, orang and gorilla. These animals, like man, have intestines eight to ten times the body length, and their diet consists of bulky food stuffs, nuts, fruits, tender shoots, juicy roots, and other vegetable foods. This is the natural diet of man, the diet of his primitive ancestors.

A bulky diet of this sort stimulates the movements of the intestine and so moves along so rapidly that there is little drying out and not sufficient time for putrefactive changes. Such a diet also insures a sufficient amount of indigestible material to distend the colon and keep its several gates in active and efficient operation.

When the diet is concentrated, leaving little residue, the residue packs firmly together, adheres to the intestine wall, gets caught in folds, and by retention becomes highly putrescent and contaminates the blood.

Another still more serious difficulty arises. As already explained, the pelvic loop, the discharging gate of the colon, collapses and falls down in the pelvis after discharging its contents. The pelvic loop remains prolapsed until it is lifted by filling. If it does not fill it does not rise and hence does not discharge, and the bowels do not move. If the food residues are so small that two days are required to supply material enough to fill the pelvic loop, then the bowel movement will occur only every other day. A water wheel will not turn without water; the colon will not act normally without the stimulus of roughage. A bulky food residue is necessary to fill and raise the pelvic loop so that it can discharge its contents.

The more bulky the diet, the more rapidly the pelvic colon will fill and the more frequently the bowels will move. The more frequent the movements, the less putrefaction and hence the less autointoxication, as shown by absence of headache, depression, coated tongue, foul breath, dingy complexion, skin troubles, chronic weariness, etc., etc.

Cellulose is the only indigestible element of the diet. Cellulose is the basis of wood; cotton is pure cellulose. Bran consists very largely of cellulose.

Starch, fat, protein, — the food materials furnished by milk, eggs, meat, fine flour bread, sugar, potatoes, and most of the breakfast foods, are completely digestible and absorbable. They disappear in the small intestine leaving no residue to fill and distend the colon and stimulate it to action. The small residues from such foods fail to fill the pelvic colon often enough to maintain frequent bowel action.

It is thus evident that we have but one alternative; we must choose our bills of fare from the coarse products on which our primitive ancestors subsisted and on which bur forest cousins still live, or we must add to our ordinary diet sufficient indigestible cellulose to supply the bulk required.

Convenient forms of cellulose are bran and agar-agar, or Japanese isinglass, a peculiar form of cellulose obtained from a sea weed which grows on the coast of Japan. One or the other of these products or combinations of the two, must be added to every meal to insure its expeditious transit along the food tube.

The idea that bran is irritating is a pernicious error. Wet bran is like wet paper, it does not and cannot irritate. Bran does not irritate the mucous membrane of the mouth. The mucous membrane of the stomach and intestine are no more sensitive nor delicate than is that of the mouth. These membranes are, in fact, less sensitive and less liable to injury than is the mouth mucosa.

Bran does not irritate, it titillates. The tongue keeps at work after a meal until every particle of food has been gathered up and disposed of. In like manner the stomach and the intestine keep at work until each little particle of bran has been passed along toward the exit.

4. *A High Protein Diet.* — By a high protein diet is meant a diet which contains an excess of the nitrogenous element of the food. Practically, such a diet will consist largely of flesh food, though an excess of protein may be taken in the form of eggs, or even in such foods as beans or certain varieties of nuts.

Man is by nature a low protein feeder. He belongs to a nut and fruit eating tribe, the primates, along with the orang and the chimpanzee. Carnivorous or flesh-eating animals have short intestines and especially very short colons.

The short intestine of the flesh-eating animal is necessary to prevent the long retention of undigested food residues. Putrefaction develops very rapidly at the temperature of the body. A bit of dead flesh in a wound soon acquires a very unpleasant odor. Even fragments of food left in the mouth in a few hours taint the breath with decomposition products. In the colon, these putrefaction changes take place much more rapidly, because of the presence of active putrefaction germs and the degree of warmth and moisture which especially favor putrefaction.

But some kinds of food do not putrefy. Practically, meat and eggs are about the only foods that undergo putrefaction or decay. Milk, cereals, vegetables, fruits, ferment, but do not putrefy. The products of fermentation are acids, chiefly lactic acid, which is non-poisonous, and even serves a useful purpose in preventing by its presence the growth of putrefaction germs and hence the decay of putrescible substances. A raw beefsteak will not decay when immersed in buttermilk or fruit juice. Sugar is a well-known preservative.

The acids formed by the fermentation of the residues of vegetable foodstuffs in the colon are the natural stimulants of the colon, an interesting fact pointed out many years ago by the eminent specialist, Prof. Ad. Schmidt.

When the fermentation is excessive, it may even give rise to looseness of the bowels as in some forms of diarrhea, in which a strong sour smell is present, common in infants.

On the other hand, putrefaction has exactly the opposite effect. The ammonia and various ptomaines and other poisons produced by the decay of meat, paralyze the colon and so cause constipation.

It is practically impossible to cure constipation so long as putrefaction is active in the colon. It should be remembered that in latent constipation there may be regular bowel movements, but the colon is never emptied. The daily evacuations represent simply the overflow of an over-distended colon filled with decaying and highly poisonous and offensive food residues.

Undigested fragments of decaying flesh are always found in the colon of meat-eaters and supply the best possible soil for the luxuriant growth of disease producing germs. Indeed, the germs which cause putrefaction, the colon bacillus, Welch's bacillus, B. putrificus and other putrefactive organisms, are all poison-forming and disease-producing germs. They cause inflammation, suppuration, abcess, gangrene, and death when their growth is unchecked. These very germs are the cause of colitis, the almost universal accompaniment of chronic constipation.

Colitis causes spasm or contraction of the lower half of the colon and exaggerated antiperistalsis, that is, reversed action of the colon, so that putrid fecal matters accumulate in the caecum, overstretch this part of the colon, and produce appendicitis, incompetency of the ileocecal valve and autointoxication.

It is evident, then, that the flesh-eating habits of Americans must be one of the great causes of the universal constipation which has become a national curse and perhaps the greatest cause of national inefficiency and physical unpreparedness.

5. *Reduced Quantity of Food.* A reduction of the quantity of food eaten lessens the bulk of the residue and so leads to constipation. Fasting, or even the omission of a meal interrupts bowel movement. Hence the need of regularity in diet. Meals must not be omitted. If there is lack of appetite or no time for the regular meal, fruit should be taken with bran or agar-agar and paraffin oil to keep up the normal rhythm, and to prevent a blockade in the lower colon.

An extra meal of fruit is an undoubted aid to bowel action. An orange or an apple eaten at bedtime is often effective in aiding the advance of the food residues so that a good evacuation is secured on rising the next morning. The activity of the colon is four times as great during the eating of food, doubtless because of the stimulating effect of food upon the controlling nerve centers through the gustatory nerves.

Even a glass or two of cold water at bed time and on rising has a similar effect. Water causes the secretion of gastric juice and excites peristaltic waves and thus aids the progress of waste along the colon.

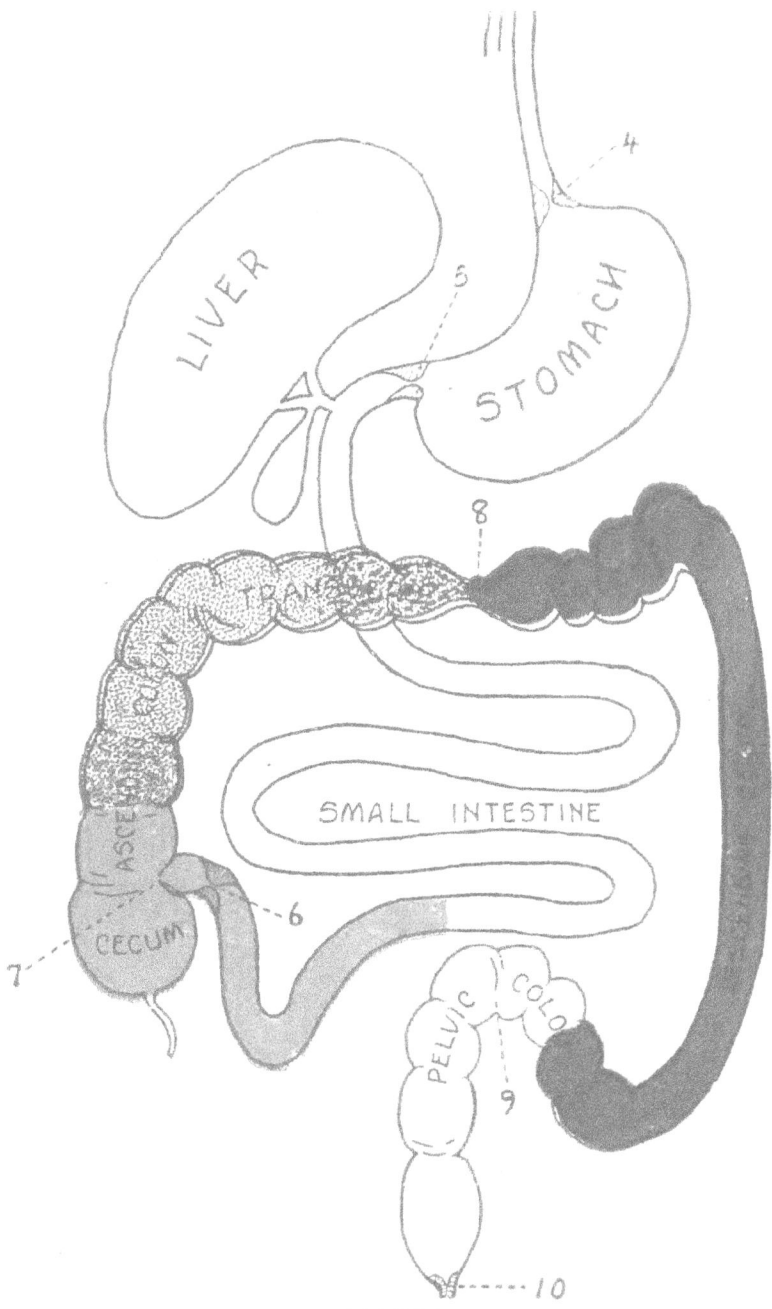

6:00 P.M.

Breakfast Residue (dark) mostly in Descending Colon.

Dinner Residue (shaded) passing into Colon, mixing with Breakfast Residue. Supper just eaten in stomach.

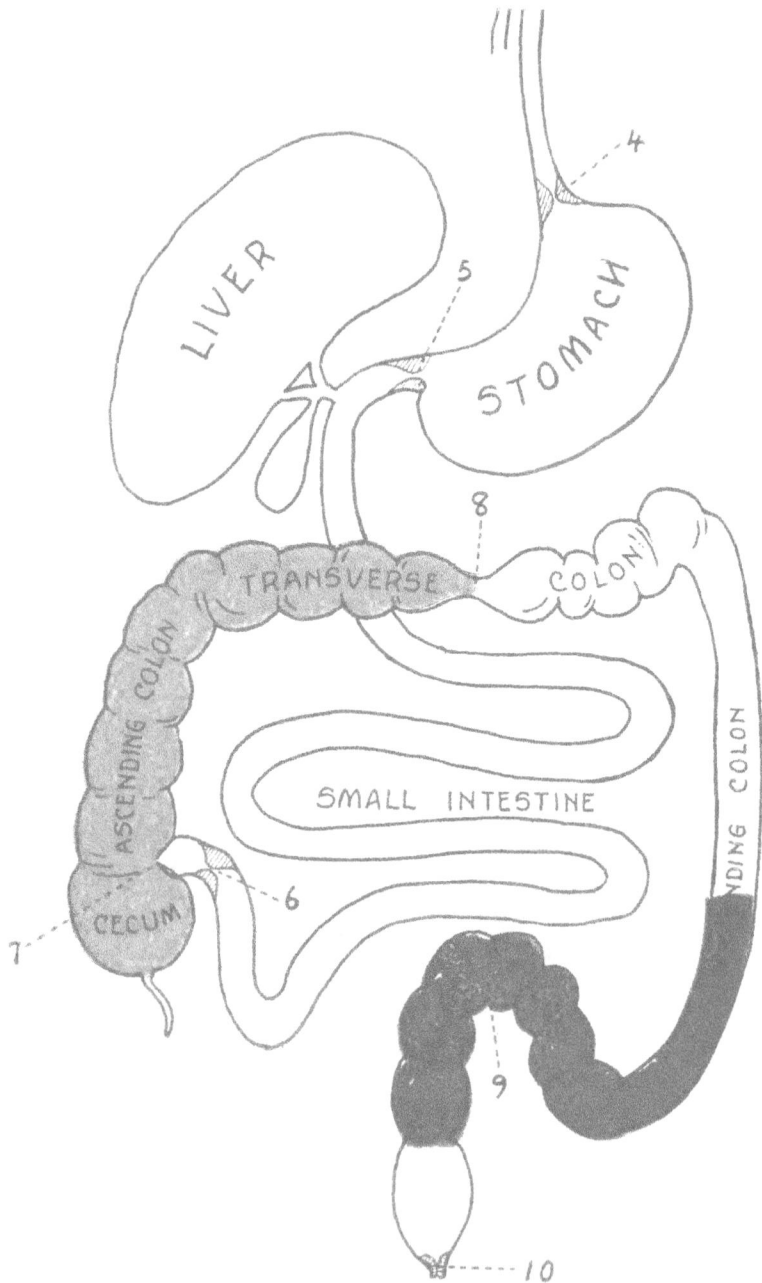

9:00 P.M.

Breakfast Residue (dark) mostly in Pelvic Colon, ready to be discharged.
Dinner Residue (shaded) in; Right Half of Colon. Supper Residue nearly ready
to enter Colon from stomach to small intestine.

Horace Fletcher's Mistake

6. It is evident that long chewing of the food must tend to aid bowel action, and that hasty eating has the opposite effect. It must be remarked, however, that by thorough mastication we do not refer to the mode of eating known as Fletcherizing. Mr. Fletcher urged that the food should be well masticated and in this many old writers as well as modern authorities are in accord with him. The writer has urged the same for more than forty years. But Mr. Fletcher also insisted that all materials which could not be reduced to a liquid in the mouth should be rejected. That is, he excluded roughage entirely from his dietary, thinking it a virtue to reduce the quantity of food residues to the smallest limit possible as a measure of economy, even to the extent of one or two bowel movements weekly. In this Mr. Fletcher was greatly in error. He evidently overlooked the fact that the body wastes which are eliminated by way of the colon are only in small part composed of food wastes, the greater and more important consisting of bile, a highly poisonous excretion, mucus, and special excretory products which are normally eliminated by way of the large intestine.

The writer labored very earnestly with Mr. Fletcher personally on many occasions to convince him of his error, and at last accounts he seems to have in some degree corrected the error as far as his own personal habits are concerned, but so far as the writer knows, he has made no attempt to correct or counteract the teaching of his books and lectures in which constipation was made to appear as a physiologic virtue, an evidence of "economy of nutrition."

This was the rock on which Fletcherism split and went to pieces as a system. It must not be forgotten, however, that Mr. Fletcher made a contribution to the science of nutrition of priceless value in compelling by his earnest and active propaganda and his tactful promotion among scientific men and physiologists, recognition of the low protein idea in diet. He went farther and contributed not much time, but many thousands of dollars to encourage scientific investigation of the question of the protein ration.

The famous research of Chittenden which demonstrated the great advantages of low protein feeding, was undertaken by the suggestion of Mr. Fletcher and the large expense was in part borne by Mr. Fletcher.

Thorough chewing, long chewing, aids the progress of food residues along the garbage canal, the colon, but only when a sufficient amount of roughage is swallowed with the digestible and nutrient portion of the foodstuffs. So one should not follow Mr. Fletcher's instruction to return to the plate everything that cannot be reduced to liquid in the mouth, but should masticate well and swallow natural food stuffs as nearly as possible in their complete entirety as nature provides them.

6. *The Educated or House-broken Colon.* — The house dog is necessarily trained to avoid evacuating his bowels in the house. In other words, he is taught to restrain his bowels from moving when they are so disposed, until it

is convenient for his owner to turn him out of doors. A dog so trained is house-broken.

If dogs were the only house-broken creatures, what a world of wretchedness, suffering, even crime and human wreckage would be saved.

All civilized people are house-broken, and like poor house-broken dogs, pay for this sinister education an infinite price, not only in misery and inefficiency, but in deadly disease and shortened life.

The whole civilized portion of the human race is house-broken. The mother or nurse of every infant begins the work of training the child to control its bowels, which means to thwart the automatic process by which the wastes are normally dismissed from the body, and by the time the child is two years old it is well house-broken and hence constipated. In this respect the infant house dog learns faster than the human infant.

A house-broken colon is a damaged colon. The natural automatic process of discarding the body wastes demands a prompt response to the "call" for evacuation. As soon as the pelvic colon, the discharging gate, is filled and lifted ready for action, a desire for evacuation is experienced. When the fecal matters begin to pass into the rectum the desire becomes so pronounced that it must be firmly resisted to avoid immediate evacuation. After a time the desire disappears, but the fecal wastes remain in the rectum. The "call" is now lost. It may return later when the rectum is still more distended by the advance into it from the pelvic colon of additional waste matters. This "call" may be resisted also, and so the rectum may become distended to the extreme limit and will no longer give notice of the entrance of feces even when it has been artificially emptied. In other words, the "call" is permanently lost, the rectum is paralyzed.

Thousands of sufferers from constipation never have a desire for evacuation except when a laxative drug has been taken.

When the call is lost, no warning is given of the condition of the colon and accumulation of waste matters may occur to an astonishing extent. Once or twice a week, perhaps, a dose of salts or of some other cathartic is taken for a sort of housecleaning and the rest of the time, filthy, putrefying wastes fill and distend the colon and cause injuries which in many instances can never be repaired.

Semi-civilized people and savages have a keen appreciation of the importance of prompt attention to the automatic demands of the body. A medical missionary who had spent many years in Arabia told the writer that a common objection offered by the tribal Arab to living in Aden was the necessity for looking up a suitable place for evacuation in compliance with the law.

A new and sensitive colon conscience must be developed among civilized people if the world is to be saved from the soul and body and even race-destroying effects of universal constipation and world wide autointoxication.

The universally prevalent idea that one bowel movement daily is sufficient is proof of the universal prevalence of constipation. One bowel movement means constipation of a pronounced degree. X-ray examination after an opaque meal shows that persons whose bowels move once a day are constantly carrying in their colons the putrefying residues of five to ten meals or even a larger number. The colon is never empty even after a movement, and toxemia is present and often shown in the coated tongue, foul breath, headache, depression, and other indications usually present.

One bowel movement a day is very marked constipation.

7. *The Use of Laxative Drugs.* — It must be admitted that the use of laxative drugs is in every way preferable to constipation. Nevertheless it must be recognized that drugs are at best only palliatives. They afford temporary relief which is sometimes highly necessary. But it must not be forgotten that at the same time they inflict grave injury upon the colon, to say nothing of injuries to the stomach, liver, kidneys and other organs, sometimes even including the heart.

Every laxative drug which acts by irritation of the colon, in time causes colitis or infection of the bowel. The congestion of the colon mucous membrane caused by the drug, destroys the filtering power of the membrane so that the poisons developed in the colon by putrefaction are readily taken into the blood, thus intensifying the effects of the intestinal toxemia always present with constipation.

Colitis is accompanied by a spastic condition of the colon. That is, the colon contracts so that the contents cannot be pushed forward *en masse*, but must be slowly carried along in lumps. The occurrence of round, hard lumps in the stool, is proof of this spastic condition. Obstructive adhesions of the pelvic colon, pouching and hindering adhesions of the caecum, incompetency of the ileocecal valve, are only a few of the mischiefs arising from the "laxative" habit.

Still another, and one of the most damaging effects of the laxative is a great exaggeration of the antiperistaltic action of the transverse colon, causing overdistension of the caecum, which in time is followed by pouching of the caecum, appendicitis and other grave conditions.

All laxative drugs are harmful. There are no exceptions. They all produce colitis and thus intensify the mischievous effects of the constipation which they temporarily remove.

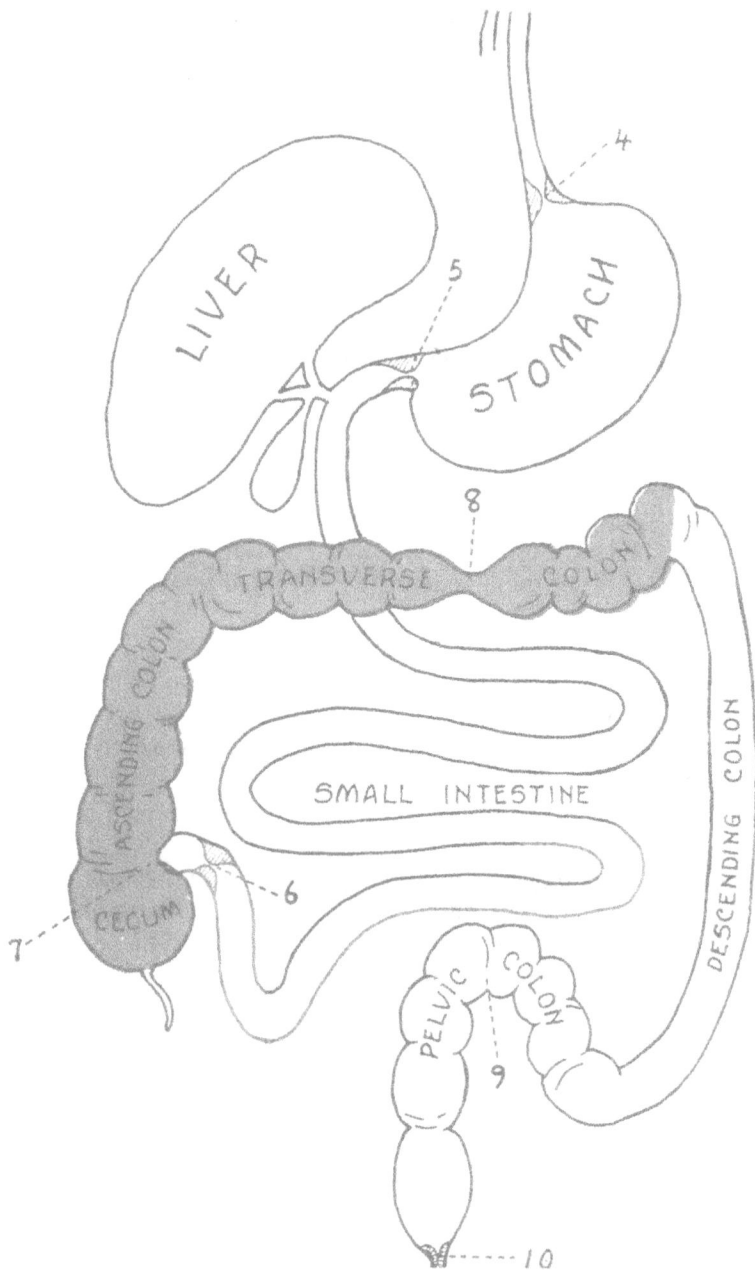

10 P.M.
Breakfast Residue (shaded) Discharged (bowel movement at bed time).
Dinner Residue in Colon, and Supper Residue ready to pass into Colon.

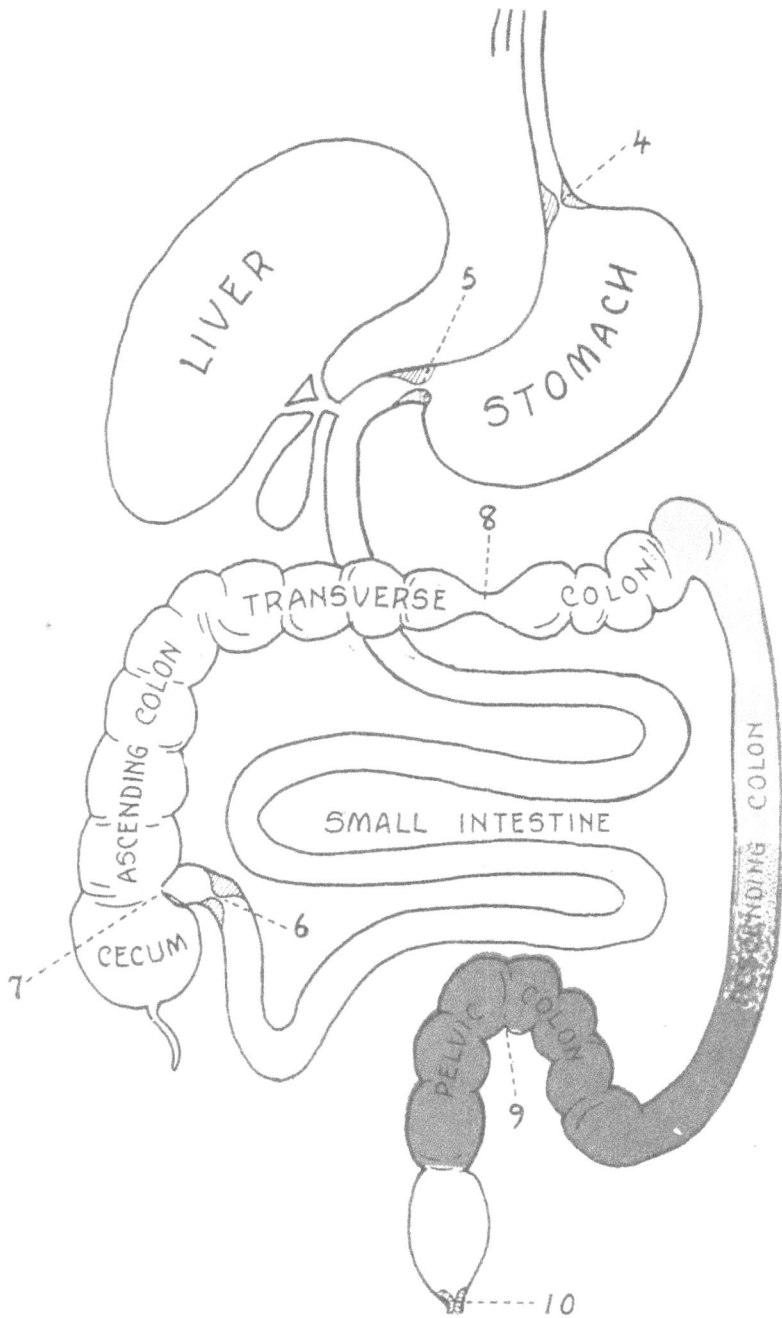

6:00 A. M.
Morning of Second Day. Dinner Residue (dark) in Pelvic Colon, ready to be discharged.

The Food Blockade

The American people are almost universally suffering from a food blockade in the colon. Constipation, the common term applied to this condition, is generally regarded as an inconvenience rather than a menace to life and health. It is one of the most prolific of all causes of disease.

Thousands of men and women think themselves in good health because their bowels move once a day, regardless of the fact that they have coated tongues, a foul breath, and many other indications of autointoxication. The fact is that the bowels should move three or four times a day — or at least once after each meal.

The normal alimentary cycle is twelve to fourteen hours. Here are the simple facts, as shown by means of X-ray examinations, experiments upon animals, and other scientific modes of investigation:

The work of digesting and absorbing the food occupies about eight hours. At the end of this time the unusable food residues is found deposited in the colon, ready to be dismissed from the body as waste and useless material. The process of gastric digestion is finished in four hours; the small intestine completes the work of digestion and absorption in four hours more.

During this time the foodstuffs have been completely digested and absorbed, or practically so, leaving a small residue of indigestible and unusable remnants, together with mucous, bile and certain other waste matters to be dismissed from the body by the colon, a wonderful mechanism provided by Nature to serve the body for waste and garbage disposal. There is in many ways close analogy between "the house we live in" and an ordinary domicile. It is almost literally true that the stomach is the kitchen of the body, the small intestine the dining room, the colon the garbage and waste disposal system — more than a mere waste receptacle.

The stomach *prepares* the food materials for digestion, but really digests and absorbs very little of the food.

The small intestine is the great digesting and absorbing department of the human economy. On its seven square feet of mucous membrane are found five millions of absorbing rootlets — the "villi" — that hang out into the cavity of the intestine. The contents of the intestine, which bathe these absorbing rootlets, constitute the soil out of which the body grows. As the soil is exhausted, the worthless remnant is pushed on into the colon, to be dismissed from the body as unusable and undesirable.

The great work of the stomach and small intestine, involving marvelous changes that fit the food to enter the blood and become part of the living structure of the body, is done in eight hours. During this time the length of intestine passed over is nearly twenty-five feet.

Clogging of the Colon

At the end of eight hours the residues are in the colon and within two or three feet of the lower outlet. If the whole mass of food, weighing several pounds in all, has been able to travel twenty-five feet in eight hours, or at the rate of three feet an hour, it certainly would seem that the small residue of waste, amounting to only a few ounces, ought to finish the journey in four hours more.

And that is exactly what occurs in the wild man who lives a natural life in the forest and in those man-like beasts, the higher apes. But among civilized people a blockade develops in this lower region of the digestive tube, which is the worse sort of obstruction to the commerce of the body and to all its activities.

X-ray studies by Dr. James T. Case have shown that the food residues of a meal reach a point beyond the middle of the colon in less than ten hours from the beginning of the meal. In two hours more, or at the end of twelve hours, these unusable materials should be cast out of the body. Certainly two hours ought to suffice for a journey of only two feet, when nearly thirty feet have been traversed in ten hours.

But the astonishing fact is that the time required for the food residues to travel the last two feet of the colon is, in the average person whose bowels move once a day, about forty hours, or twenty times longer than it should be.

In this astonishing fact is to be found the secret of nine-tenths of all the chronic ills from which civilized human beings suffer, and perhaps not a small part of our moral and social maladies.

In the last two feet of the colon is found the seat of the most destructive blockade that has ever opposed human progress. Let us look a moment at the real situation. The accompanying diagrams will help to make this clear. (See colored plates.)

Suppose a test meal is given at breakfast on Monday morning. Within the fifty or more hours that elapse before the residues of the meal are dismissed on the following Wednesday, at least six more meals are eaten. The residues of all these meals as well as those of the test meal are packed away in the co-lon. The residue of the test meal is shown in the accompanying colored dia-grams in black. The succeeding meal residues are shown in red, blue and yel-low colors.

How far different this condition is from a normal or ideal state will best be appreciated by reference to the second diagram. When the colon acts nor-mally the food residues are moved along in a procession with intervals be-tween the meals which afford the intestine an opportunity for rest, and, still more important, a chance to cleanse itself by means of its lubricating and disinfecting mucus. Each residue should be moved along by itself and dis-charged at once when it reaches the end of the colon. Here is the normal pro-gram of the procession along the food tube:

Breakfast at 7 a.m.

At 11 a. m. the stomach is empty and has an opportunity to rest and disinfect itself before dinner. The breakfast is all in the small intestine and beginning to pass into the colon.

Dinner at noon.

The new peristaltic impulse given the whole food tube by the new intake of food carries the breakfast over into the colon and by five o'clock p. m. the breakfast has begun to enter the descending or last half of the colon, the dinner is in the lower part of the small intestine, and the stomach is again empty, resting and disinfecting itself in preparation for supper.

Supper at 6 p.m.

The new food intake makes another vigorous move all along the line, the result of which in four hours should be to dismiss the whole residue of the breakfast, to move the dinner residue into the colon, and to carry the supper to the lower end of the small intestine, leaving the stomach empty and so prepared for rest during the night.

During the hours of sleep the intestinal movements are much slower. By morning however, the dinner residue of the day before will have reached the lower colon, so that the intestinal activity set up by the act of rising should lead to a before breakfast bowel movement.

The breakfast intake should cause the dismissal of the residue of the supper of the day before; or if the after-breakfast movement fails or is incomplete, the dinner intake should lead to a complete clearance of all the residues accumulated from the food intakes of the day before.

When this program is carried out without interruption, no part of the food tube is over-burdened with an undue accumulation of waste material, and the food residues are moved along so rapidly that there is no time for harmful putrefaction.

It is known that the first changes that occur in the foodstuffs are simple acid fermentations that are harmless. It is only after the lapse of twenty-four hours or more that putrefaction and poison-forming processes begin. It is thus evident that the maintenance of the normal alimentary cycle is a matter of the utmost consequence for health preservation, and that the restoration of this function when lost is a matter of fundamental importance.

X-ray studies have clearly shown that in by far the great majority of cases of constipation, perhaps in nine-tenths of all cases, the real difficulty is to be found in the lower part of the colon.

A common and most valuable remedy which has been resorted to even by the most primitive people and from the most ancient times, is the enema, by which the crippled colon is mechanically emptied. This harmless measure affords only temporary relief, and to be effective must be repeated daily, and twice a day when natural movements do not occur without.

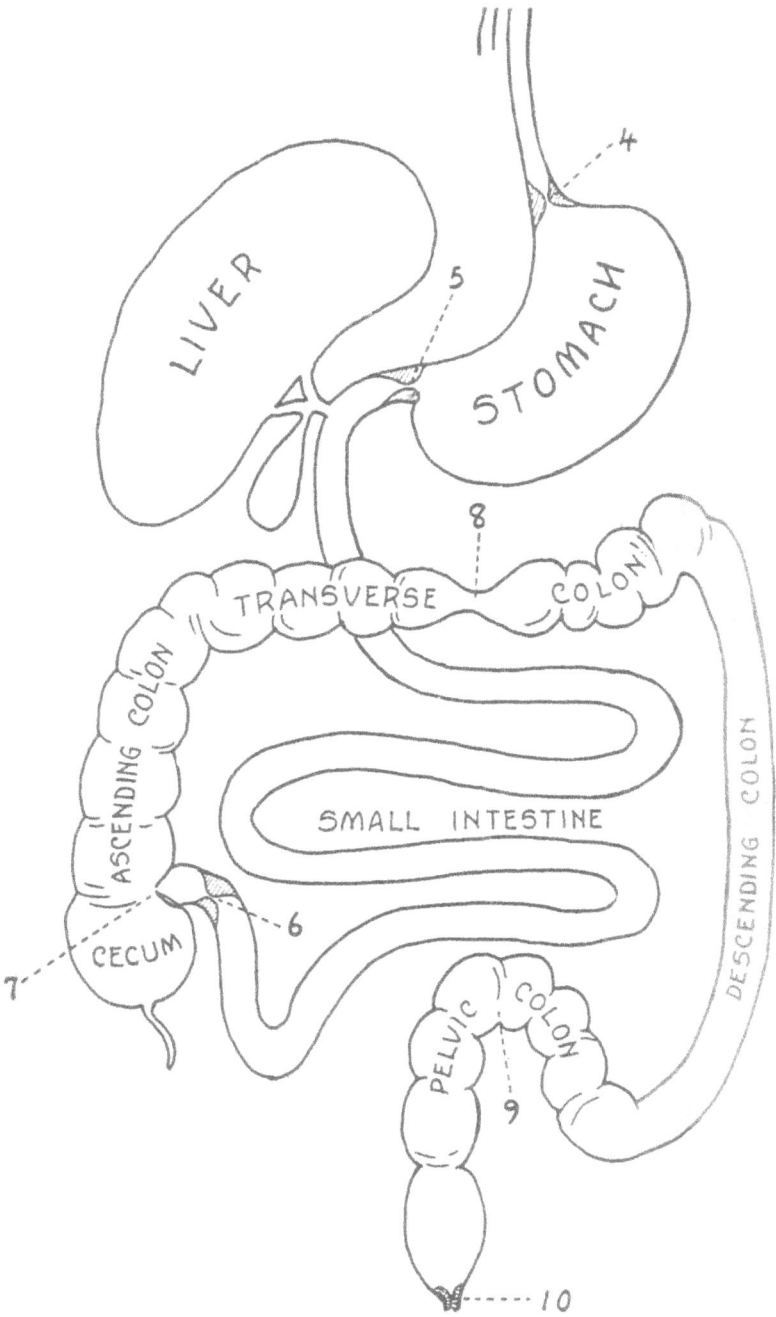

6:30 A.M.
Half Hour after Rising, Second Day, after Bowel Movement. Only Residue of Supper left in descending Colon.

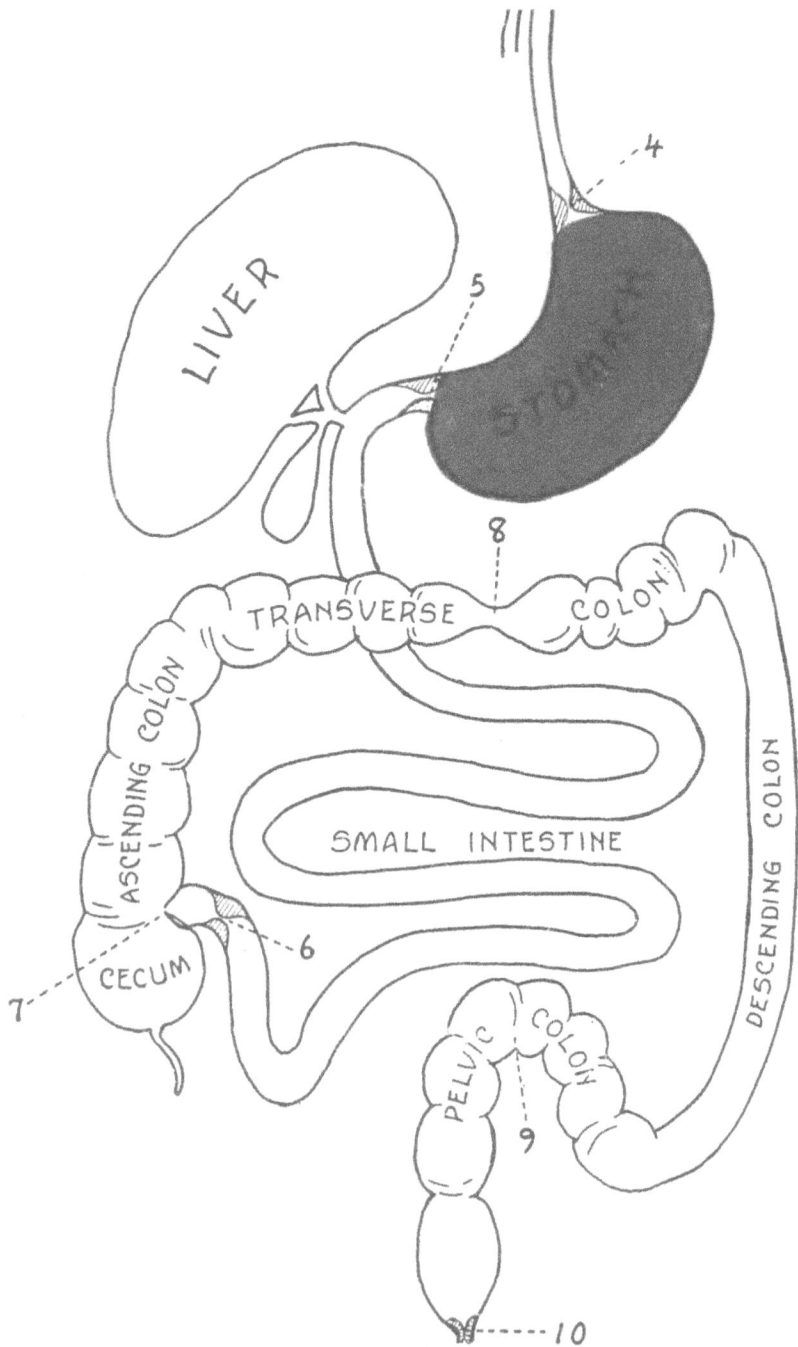

8:00-9:00 A. M. (Second Day)

Second Morning after Breakfast. Bowels have moved, the Colon has been emptied of wastes and residue, and is ready for a new series of meals.

Bulk and Lubrication

The most valuable, remedies, measures that actually succeed, even in very obstinate cases, are found in two very simple substances — bran and paraffine oil. One affords bulk, the other lubrication.

By the proper use of bran, or agar-agar, and paraffine oil at each meal, the bowels may be made to move normally, or at least in a manner approximating the normal rhythm — that is, three times a day, or after each meal. The amount of bran or other bulk material must be large, two ounces daily being required in some cases.

The amount of paraffine required also differs. In some cases the dose must be quite large — even so much as an ounce and a half at each meal. The amount of bran and paraffine should be gradually increased until sufficient to accomplish its purpose.

How to Raise the Blockade

When the tongue is coated and the breath bad, it is well to begin the battle for raising the blockade with a few days of fruit regimen. This consists of a dietary composed wholly of fruits, with bran and paraffine. Under this regimen the tongue becomes clean, the breath sweet and the bowels move three or four times a day. By careful management of the diet, this improved condition may be rendered permanent, but a never-ending battle must be waged against constipation. The colon is crippled and will always need special attention and help. It has become overstretched and half paralyzed, and so an extra amount of roughage or bulk-making material in the shape of fruits, vegetables, bran or agar-agar will always be needed. The mucous glands have atrophied and perhaps the appendix has been removed, and so the lubricating system of the intestine is damaged, and it may be necessary to make permanent use of an artificial lubricant — paraffine oil in some form. *Bulk and lubrication must be provided for every meal.*

The Crippled Colon

Crippled colons may be responsible for half the ills of life. They are the cause of most of the headaches, the insomnia, depression, nerves, neuralgia, hypochondria and "biliousness," to say nothing of neuritis, rheumatism, and a score of other painful or dangerous maladies. Many diseases, the origin of which has long been a mystery, are now believed by able physicians to be due to the poisons generated by putrefactive processes in the colon.

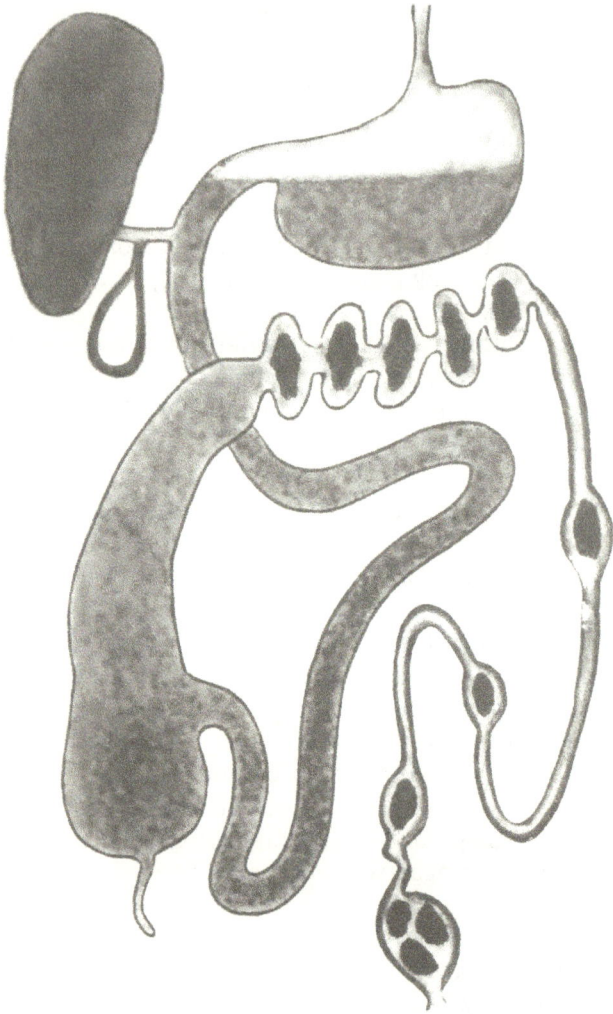

A Crippled Colon

Diagram showing the condition of the colon in chronic constipation as revealed by the X-ray. Spastic contraction of the colon due to colitis. Dilated cecum, incompetent ileocecal valve, ileac and gastric stasis, inflammation of gall-bladder.

Colon Hygiene

We hear much nowadays about the hygiene of the mouth, and the newspapers teem with wise and unwise advice about the care of the stomach, but rarely do we hear anything really helpful or sensible about the hygiene of the colon, the terminal portion of the alimentary canal.

The mouth is the receiving station, the colon is the waste disposal plant. The wastes with which the colon deals are only in part composed of food residues. The larger part consists of bile, mucus and other body wastes, poisonous matters which must be eliminated in order to keep the blood clean and the body free from hindering refuse.

The mismanagement of the receiving station is a prolific source of trouble and of disease. This every one knows, most people from personal experience. Not so many people are aware of the fact that a still longer list of ills and still more serious disorders result from derangements of the waste disposal plant. When the food residues, and other wastes, are not promptly dismissed from the body they undergo putrefaction. This is the cause of the extremely offensive character of the fecal matters, especially the bowel discharges of dogs, cats, lions, and other animals that eat meat. The undigested portion of meat undergoing decay in the colon gives rise to the same obnoxious odors and the same rank poisons which are found in a dead rat or the carcass of a dead cow decaying in a fence corner.

It is necessary to take in food at frequent intervals. It is equally necessary to dispose of the food residues and body wastes at frequent intervals. The kidneys remove poisons which are temporarily deposited in the bladder and discharged several times a day. The liver excretes daily twenty ounces of bile which, according to Bouchard, is six times as poisonous as urine, and this needs to be discharged along with other wastes as promptly and as frequently as is the urine. In other words, it is just as important that the colon should be emptied several times a day as that the bladder should be emptied several times daily. In fact, the bowels should be emptied at least after every meal.

Bowel Habits of Wild Animals, Wild Men and Idiots

Wild animals, wild men, healthy infants and idiots move their bowels as often as they are fed. Wild animals and wild men have better sense than to interfere with the normal promptings of nature. Infants and idiots lack the intelligence necessary to disturb their normal functions, and so the bowels move automatically soon after food is taken. In well-managed idiot asylums the inmates are regularly taken to the toilet after each meal and before going to bed. When this is done, the soiling of beds and clothing is prevented.

When the colon acts in this prompt and regular way, there is little time for the putrefaction of food residues in the colon, and the stools are less offensive, especially when meat is excluded from the dietary.

Injurious Conventionalities

Most civilized human beings, and sometimes pet animals, are less fortunate than wild animals, wild men and idiots in relation to their bowel functions. Almost from the first dawn of intelligence the infant is systematically taught to restrain its bowel and bladder functions. The demands of modesty and our ignorance of the importance of frequent, rhythmical and automatic bowel action lead to restraint, delay, and neglect of the body's waste disposal function to such a degree as to make it an actual menace to the welfare of the race.

A Lesson from an Idiot Asylum

Miss Keller, an inspector connected with the health department of New York city, sent the author the following highly interesting observation respecting the bowel habits of idiots which must of necessity be automatic, and hence more likely to be natural than the habits of those whose intelligence permits them in obedience to the mandates of pernicious custom to ignore and set aside the warning of nature, and to thwart and finally destroy important automatic functions:

"The following observation may interest you. It was made while inspecting Randall's Island's Children's Hospitals and Schools, the place where New York City maintains its feeble-minded public charges, about two thousand in number, who range from rank idiocy through imbecility and up to the moron grade. There are also a few epileptics.

"In looking into sanitary conditions, and finding both the inmates and the premises clean, I asked the matron in charge of one cottage harboring one hundred and eighty-six children of the lowest type of mentality, how she managed to keep them continent. She said the children are trained to evacuate their bowels four times each day, once after each meal and once before bedtime. Those whose mentality is too low to form the habit of going to the toilet are placed on it by attendants. The others are directed there after meals. The results are quite mechanical.

"It was interesting to note how many of those who have been there for some time have clear looking skins and eyes, while many of the new arrivals are sallow and have pimpled skins."

Instead of training the child to restrain its functions, to resist the call to nature for the evacuation of poisonous wastes, it should be taught that these functions are of greatest importance and that the demand of nature should be respected and should receive immediate attention. To protect the child from embarrassment and to ensure normal functioning, the child should be trained from earliest years to visit the toilet at once after each meal, before going to bed, and on rising in the morning.

No possible harm can come from these frequent bowel movements, and when the diet is properly regulated, no difficulty will be experienced in establishing good bowel habits, especially if the instruction is begun early and if there is never any interruption of the normal bowel rhythm.

The neglect of the colon is so common among civilized people that constipation has become an almost universal condition. It is, indeed, so common that a wholly wrong conception of the bowel function has become current. It is almost universally believed by physicians, as well as laymen, that one bowel movement a day is quite sufficient to meet natural requirements and "a well-formed stool" is the evidence of perfect "regularity."

Interesting Japanese Colon Customs

The Japanese are an exceedingly practical people, and, although rapidly becoming sophisticated are not yet so far away from the influence of their primitive life as to have become obtuse to their physical needs as are the people of the older civilizations. A highly intelligent American lady who has lived long in Japan and become very intimately acquainted with the habits and manners of the people, has given me the following most interesting account of the very sensible manner in which the Japanese deal with matters pertaining to the evacuation of wastes: —

"The Japanese show no false modesty whatever in answering the call of nature. For no matter what the time, place or circumstances may be, they do not hesitate to excuse themselves and go to the toilet whenever they experience a "call."

"The guests who visit us in our home, even the gentlemen callers, think no more of asking where the toilet is than of speaking of the weather.

"In most of the houses of the Japanese there are two toilets, one very near the reception room and the other nearer the living rooms of the family.

"If you are a guest in a friend's home and must go to the toilet, you cannot possibly avoid observation for the toilet is in plain view.

"The toilets themselves are different from ours in that there is no stool or chair but simply a hole in the floor over a large jar so that in evacuating the bowels one assumes a squatting position, and the children are taught from babyhood up to press the knees against the abdomen when evacuating the bowels.

"As to the convenient location of toilets, they are not only in every railway station, public building, etc., but on the corner of every block or two in all the cities and towns. These public toilets the natives use freely.

"As to their diet, not until the white man came into their country and taught them to do so, did they eat meat of any kind except fish.

Even now in some of the Buddhist sects the eating of the flesh of animals, except fish, is prohibited.

"In the interior, most of the housewives know nothing of how to kill and dress a chicken, and in our cooking classes for the women they beg us to teach them how to fry a beefsteak and they think that we have meat at every meal and many different kinds at each meal.

"They eat a great many different kinds of vegetables, especially greens of all kinds and seaweed (agar-agar) is a favorite dish. Fruit is served at every meal. After a feast the last thing served is not coffee but fruit.

"The Japanese say that we, the white man, have a peculiar odor about us which is to them very offensive, and that this odor is due to the eating of the flesh of fowls and beasts."

The above most interesting observations very fully confirm the author's views respecting the normal intestinal rhythm when the automatic mechanism devised by nature for the evacuation of the body wastes is allowed to operate without interference by voluntary restraint.

One Daily Evacuation Is Chronic Constipation

The truth is, one bowel movement a day is serious constipation, and a "well-formed stool" is absolute proof of stagnation of the colon contents and autointoxication. When the bowels move with normal frequency there is not time for the food residues to become dried out and molded into a semi-solid mass.

X-ray examinations of the alimentary tract have shown that when the bowels move but once daily, the residues of a test meal are not fully discharged until the third day, or fifty hours or more from the time the meal was taken. It is evident that in such cases not only the residues of the test meal are in the colon but also that the residues of all the meals taken after the test meal during the two days. That is, besides the test meal (breakfast) residues there are the residues of the dinner and supper of the same day and the breakfast, dinner, and supper of the next day, five meals in addition to the test meal.

This is the constant situation with a person whose bowels move once a day. When the bowels move naturally only every other day, or when stimulated by a laxative, the situation is very much worse. In such cases the colon often contains the residues of a dozen meals or more.

When the bowels move normally after each meal there is never found In the body at one time more than three meal residues and nothing remains in the colon longer than twenty-four hours. It is probable that the normal motility period of the human alimentary canal is ten to fourteen hours. That is, the residue of the breakfast should be dismissed before bedtime, the residue of dinner on rising next morning, and the supper residue after breakfast or dinner.

It is not to be expected that this ideal condition can be established in all cases, nor even in the majority of cases of chronic constipation, because in these obstinate cases the colon has become so badly crippled, the delicate nerves and muscular machinery, by which the food residues and body wastes are disposed of have been so greatly damaged, that the best results that can be hoped for are only an approximation to normal conditions.

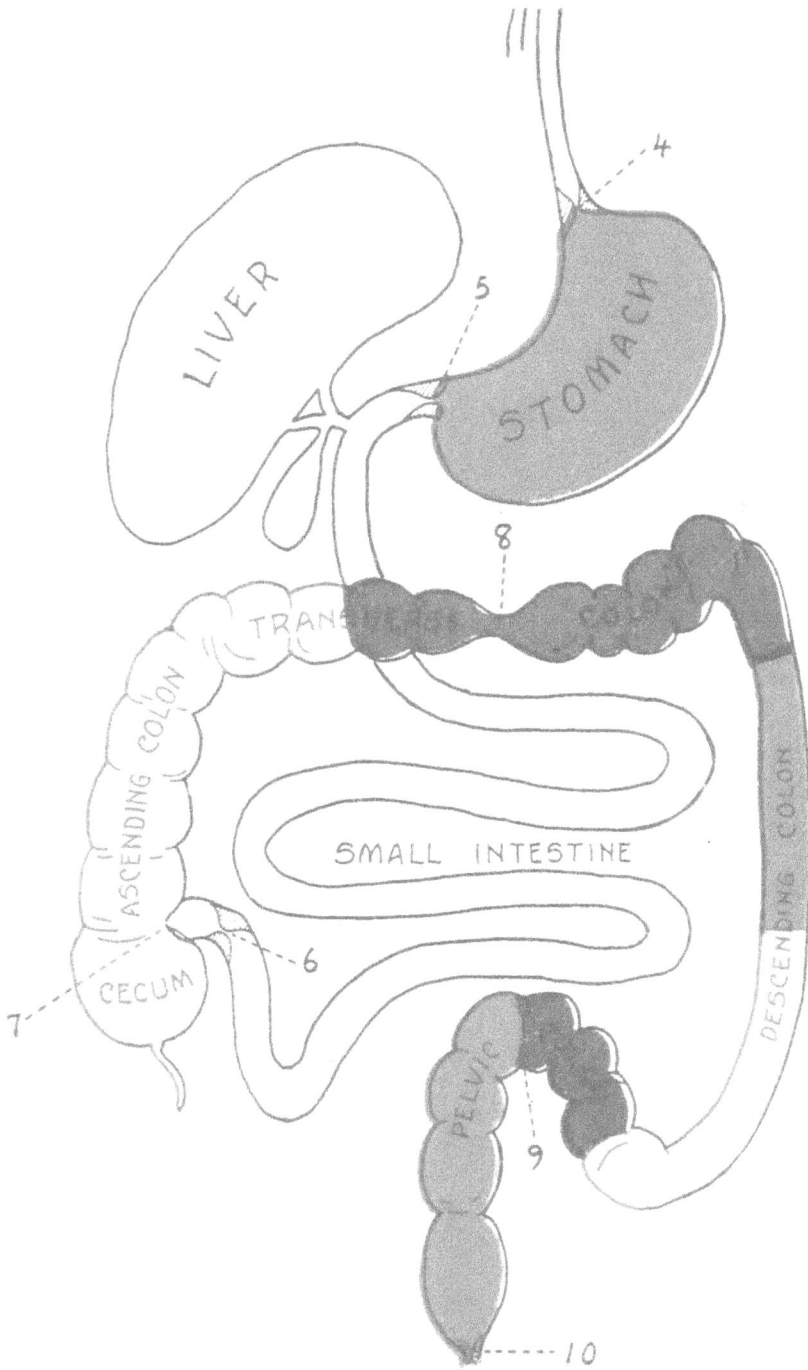

Diagram Showing Condition of the Colon when the Bowels Move once Daily,
containing the Residues of Six Meals.

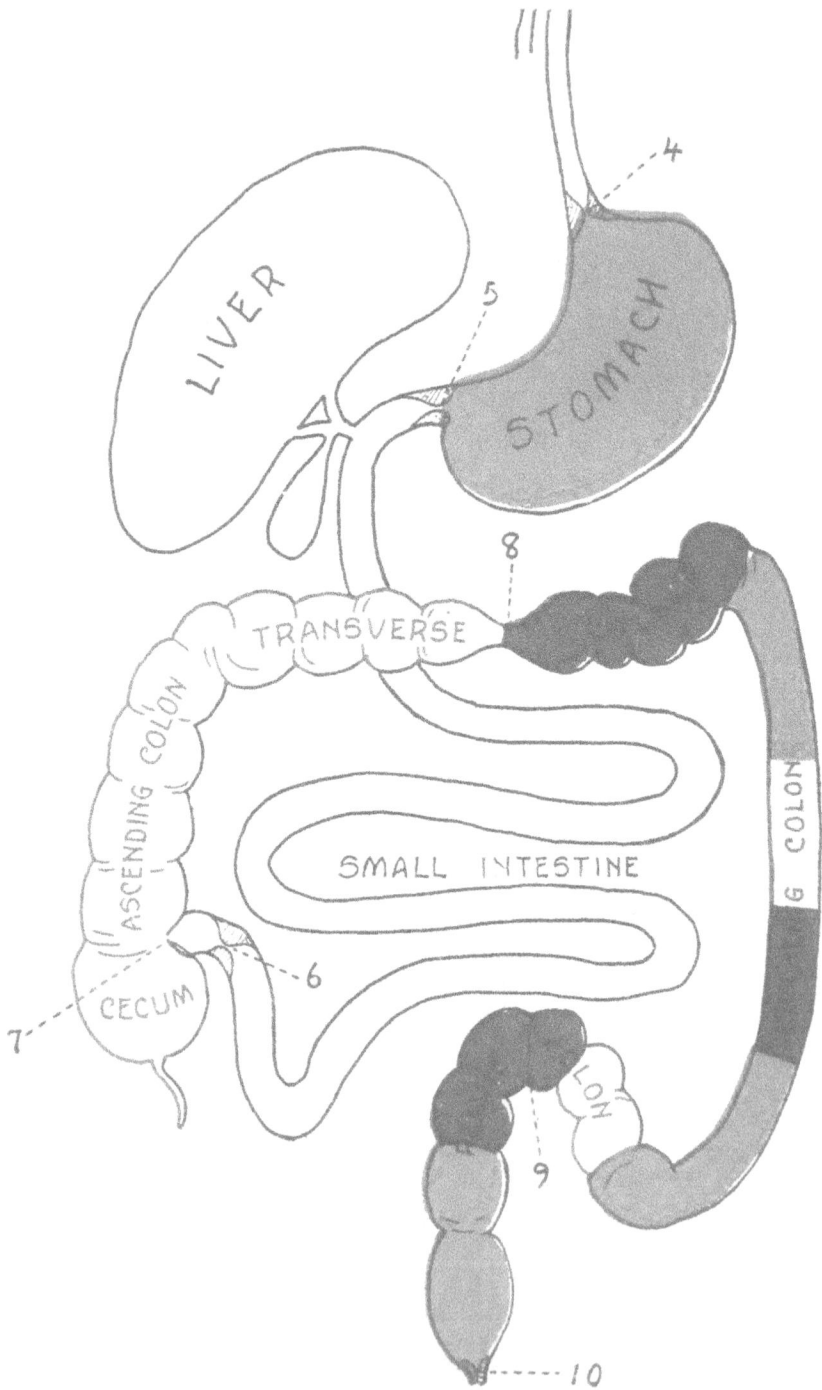

Diagram Showing Condition of the Colon in Chronic Constipation, containing the Residues of Nine or more Meals.

Abnormal Colon Conditions

The diseased conditions which are most commonly involved in constipation are the following:

1. *Paralysis of the rectum* from resisting the promptings of nature. The "call" has been lost by neglect.

Normally, the rectum is highly sensitive. It is empty except during bowel movement. As soon as a small amount of fecal matter enters the upper part of the rectum, a desire for evacuation is experienced. While this sensation calls attention to the need for evacuation the same nerve stimulation operates a reflex by which the colon is made to contract and empty itself if given an opportunity to do so. If, however, the "call" is resisted, the sensation ceases, the rectum becomes filled with fecal matters but gives no sign of their presence. The rectum becomes greatly distended and is really paralyzed.

This is rectal constipation and is by far the most common sort. It is the natural consequence of neglect. Fortunately, rectal constipation is always curable, but very thoroughgoing and prolonged treatment is required.

The rectum must be kept empty by the aid of the cool enema (80°-70°F) twice a day. Paraffin oil in some form, bran, or agar-agar and a laxative diet must be consistently adhered to. Electricity is often useful in restoring normal sensibility.

Regular times for evacuation are highly important. An effort should be made after each meal. The aid of the cool enema may be resorted to with benefit in many cases to initiate the normal habit of evacuating after every meal.

2. *A contracted or "tight" anal sphincter* may be the cause of delayed movements and rectal constipation.

When ulcers, hemorrhoids, or other painful conditions of the rectum exist, or "tight" sphincter, the anal sphincter should be stretched and proper surgical treatment applied.

3. *Colitis.* — A spastic contraction, or cramp of the bowel, occurs in colitis, causing obstinate constipation so-called, "spastic constipation. Hot fomentations to the abdomen and the warm enema will temporarily relax the spasm, but the colitis must be cured by changing the intestinal flora, that is, driving out the putrefactive bacteria and establishing the protective acid-forming germs, which not only prevent putrefaction, but by means of the acids which they produce stimulate the bowel to normal activity. The ammonia and other bases caused by putrefaction paralyze the colon. Colitis is always curable by use of modern scientific methods.

4. *Prolapse of the pelvic colon*, the last loop of the bowel, is a very common cause of obstinate constipation. When adhesions have formed, an operation is sometimes necessary. The pelvic colon must rise as it fills to enable it to empty itself naturally.

5. *Adhesions of the caecum.* — The head of the caecum receives the food residues from the small intestine and should be able to contract so as to push

its contents up and around the liver angle of the colon. When the csecum is adherent it cannot contract and the residues accumulate in the bowel and only move along the colon as pushed forward by accumulating material continually entering from the small intestine.

6. *Adhesions of the appendix* bind and cripple the colon the same as adhesions of the caecum. This is perhaps the reason why chronic appendicitis is always accompanied by constipation. Persons who have been operated for appendicitis usually suffer from constipation perhaps because of adhesions of the caecum resulting from the operation.

7. *A dilated or a pouched caecum* is equally crippling. The over-stretched bowel loses its contractile power.

It is to be remembered also that the appendix is an important part of the lubricating system of the colon. The loss of the abundant supply of lubricating mucus which it normally furnishes may be a cause of constipation.

Constipation of a very obstinate sort is found in most cases in which the appendix has been removed or in which it is the subject of chronic disease. In such cases the colon is permanently crippled by the loss of this very essential feature of its lubricating mechanism.

In such a caecal pouch putrid matters accumulate and become extremely virulent. The caecum becomes a sort of cesspool in which decomposable residues may remain for several days or longer.

A proper change in diet and special measures of various sort greatly improve this condition but in many cases it is necessary to wash out the colon by means of an enema daily or at least every other day. These cases are not relieved by laxatives. The enema is the only unfailing method. The daily use of the cool enema is not in any way injurious and may be continued indefinitely without harm.

8. *An incompetent ileocecal valve* is both a consequence and a cause of constipation. This interesting structure acts as a check valve and thus makes possible the uniform advancement of the bowel content. When the valve is broken down and incompetent the material which enters the colon from the small bowel returns to the small intestine when the bowel contracts, and surges back and forth without making definite progress. Gases are especially troublesome. When the colon contracts, its contents are expelled at both ends, at the lower externally, at the upper into the small bowel.

Tumors, cancer, adhesions and obstructive "kinks" are other recognized but rare causes of obstinate constipation.

Fortunately, this long list of colon conditions is really **not so formidable as it looks**. Two very simple remedies will almost always accomplish a cure. These are bulk and lubrication. The bulk is found in sterilized bran or agar-agar; the lubrication in paraffin oil. These remedies must be systematically used, at every single meal, unfailingly, and in such quantity as may be needed to produce the results required. Large amounts are sometimes necessary at first.

It is highly important to have an X-ray examination of the colon made in all cases of obstinate constipation so that the exact condition present may be discovered. With this highly important knowledge in his possession, the up-to-date physician is now able to deal successfully with practically every case of constipation. Operation is sometimes required, but only in very rare cases.

X-Ray Views of the Food Tube

Since scientific observation has fixed the normal time for the food transit and has worked out the actual time table so that we know when the food or food residues of a meal should arrive at each particular station, it becomes a matter of great interest to have some method by means of which we may check up the progress of a meal along the food tube and note the time of arrival at the different stations and the time occupied by the whole journey from the entrance to exit, the so-called "motility period." This has come to be a matter of the greatest moment since we have been made acquainted by Metchnikoff, Bouchard and others, with the terrible consequences which result from delay at way stations, through the putrefaction of food residues, secretions, wastes and partly digested food stuffs.

Modern science has provided two methods of studying "motility" which are capable of rendering the most signal service. These are the X-ray test meal and the color test.

X-Ray Study of Motility

This test is based upon the fact that certain substances are opaque to the X-rays and cause them to show a shadow on a specially prepared screen or on a photographic plate.

The most elaborate and complete method of X-ray examination of the colon was devised by Dr. James T. Case, roentgenologist of the Battle Creek Sanitarium, who is now Lieut. Colonel of the U. S. Army, Senior Consultant in Roentgenology for the American Expeditionary force in France, to whom the world is greatly indebted for many important observations and discoveries in connection with the X-ray study of the stomach and colon.

What the X-Ray Expert Sees

An X-ray examination of a person without special preparation would usually show very little respecting the stomach or intestine for the reason that these parts are practically transparent to the X-rays. Special preparation of the subject must be made. This special preparation consists of two things; comlete emptying of the stomach and intestine and second, the giving to the patient of a special meal, which usually consists of a pint of gruel of some sort or a couple of glasses of buttermilk to which has been added an ounce or two of bismuth or barium in fine powder.

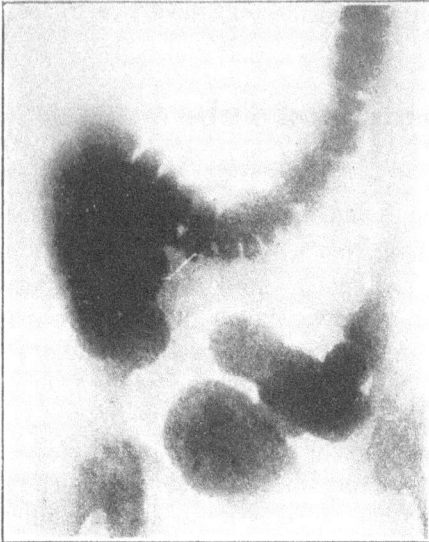

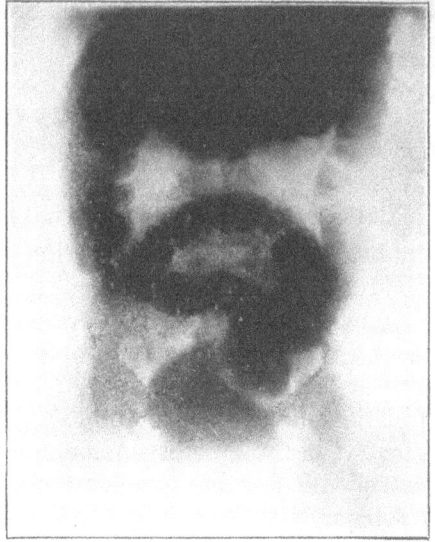

Adherent Pelvic Colon   Pelvic Colon Restored to Position by Operation

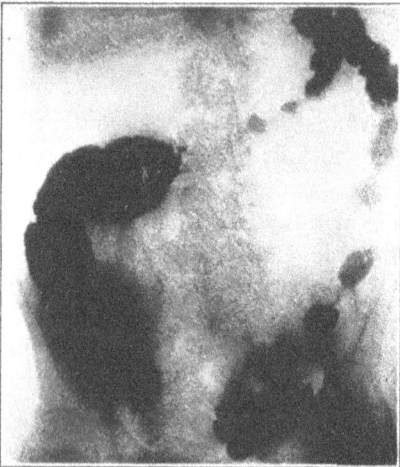

Reverse Peristalsis   Incompetent Heocecal Valve

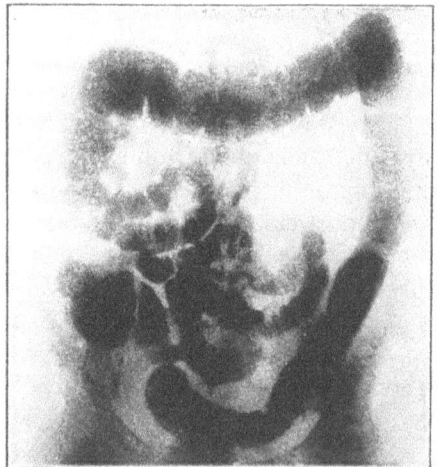

These mineral substances, as well as others, are opaque to the X-ray. That is, they cast a shadow. The stomach and intestines being hollow organs, the shadow formed by the opaque meal takes the form of the stomach or of that part of the intestine in which it appears.

When a person who has taken an opaque meal is placed in the X-ray apparatus, the shadow of the meal is thrown upon a screen under the eye of the observer, who is thus able to note the location of the meal, the form of the part in which it is located and to compare it with the normal, and likewise to observe the changes in form and location which are always taking place.

The observer begins his examination by placing the subject between 'the X-ray tube and a fluorescent screen and seats himself upon a stool in front of the screen. The subject is now given the test meal, and as he swallows it the expert watches the behavior of the stomach as each morsel enters. In health, everything proceeds in the most orderly fashion. As one morsel succeeds another, it passes along a definite course until it reaches a state of rest and is lost in the accumulating mass.

The reception of food into the stomach starts up a series of movements which should proceed in a definite and well-known order. Any deviation from the normal standard is quickly noted and recorded.

The stomach movements are not so rapid, however, that the X-ray cannot catch them on the screen and record them on a photographic plate.

The observer notes with the greatest care the behavior of the stomach as the food passes out of the pylorus and of the small intestine, the duodenum, as the food enters it. The action of the pylorus is watched with special care since it is at or near this point that many of the most troublesome changes in the stomach occur. There may be deformities due to ulcer or cancer, obstruction, or other departures from the normal.

The duodenum is carefully scrutinized for the presence of ulcer or adhesions which may obstruct or delay the passage of food through it.

After a thorough initial scrutiny the subject is released and asked to return at stated intervals during the day when the observations made show the progress of the test meal along the road from stomach to colon.

The observations are renewed the next day, at less frequent intervals, to note the length of time the food residues remain in the colon and any obstructive conditions that may exist.

The ileocecal valve, the caecum, the appendix, the several parts of the colon, ascending, transverse, descending, and pelvic colon and the rectum, all are carefully inspected. By means of pressure applied at various points the absence or presence of adhesions is determined. When adhesions are present, the mobility of the various organs is lessened; that is, they cannot be moved about as freely as in normal conditions. For example, when ulcers of the duodenum of a serious character are present, it is not uncommon for the X-ray expert to find adhesions about the duodenum which bind the duodenum and restrict the mobility of the stomach. In chronic inflammation of the gall-bladder, the adjacent parts, stomach, liver, duodenum, and gall-bladder, and sometimes the colon and other parts are very likely to be bound tightly together by adhesions.

The small intestines, the caecum, the appendix, the transverse colon, and the pelvic colon are also studied with great care with reference to adhesions, which in these parts are often the source of great mischief and chronic disorders, especially autointoxication from most obstinate constipation.

The size and form of the various parts of the colon are of great significance and are most carefully noted as well as the position of the several parts. The accompanying cuts show better than any description some of the various wonderful things which a really expert roentgenologist is able to see by means of the X-ray.

The patient is examined at stated intervals until the last trace of bismuth has disappeared from the alimentary tract. Sometimes a diseased appendix retains traces of bismuth for several days after it has disappeared from other parts.

Finally a bismuth enema is given while the expert watches the behavior of the colon as the enema enters. This part of the examination is highly important as it may reveal the presence of cancer or adhesions or other causes of mechanical obstruction, as well as deformities of the gut, pouches, dilations, "kinks," etc. and in many cases incompetency of the ileocecal valve.

Besides these "fleuroscopic" observations, plates are made, roentgenograms, which reveal some things not otherwise discoverable, and form a permanent record.

The information which may be obtained by a careful X-ray study of the interior of the body, especially of the abdomen, is often of greater importance and value than what might be learned by opening the abdomen and viewing the parts with the eye. The X-ray gives information about conditions which are beyond the reach of the eye even with the organs in sight.

But emphasis should be laid upon the fact that an X-ray apparatus alone is not sufficient to secure useful information. A well-trained X-ray expert as well as an up-to-date apparatus must be on the job.

The X-ray only makes shadows. The expert must interpret the shadows. Long years of training and education of the eye to observe fine distinctions of light and shade, and deep study of physiology and pathology as well as of the physics and the technic of the X-ray are essential to success. Only such an expert can be trusted.

A tyro misinterprets what he sees. The minute indications of disease he overlooks, and unusual but perfectly normal appearances he mistakes for cancer or some other dreadful condition for which he urges immediate operation.

Unfortunately the country is full of X-ray tyros, thanks to the commercial activity of X-ray machine manufacturers. It is safe to say that at the present moment the conclusions drawn from the majority of X-ray examinations of the colon are altogether unreliable and worthless, if not positively misleading, and a menace to the patient's welfare if made a basis for active treatment or operation.

Beware of the X-ray tyro. There are in the United States possibly one hundred X-ray specialists whose examinations of the alimentary canal may be regarded as of value and whose conclusions may be trusted as fairly reliable; but the chances are very great that our estimate is far too large.

A Simple "Motility" Test

The time which elapses after a test meal is taken before the discharge of the indigestible residues is termed the motility period of the food tube, that is, the time required for the complete journey from entrance to exit.

Several writers have placed the motility period at fifty hours. It is evident, however, that these authorities were dealing with constipated persons, those whose bowels move once a day. When the bowels move in a normal manner, or three or four times daily, the motility period is shortened. In the writer's opinion, 24 to 25 hours should be regarded as the outside limit for normal motility, and really normal bowel activity, as elsewhere observed, may be reckoned as 14 to 16 hours.

Thousands of persons whose bowels move daily would be surprised to find on examination of their motility a period of two to three days or even more. Not infrequently the period is lengthened to five or six days.

The value of this information is so great that in the writer's opinion every adult person should have the test applied, especially if at all constipated.

Fortunately we are in possession of a very simple and efficient means of applying the test. A capsule containing fifteen grams of carmine is swallowed just before breakfast. At each bowel movement thereafter the color is observed. The time is noted when the red color is first seen and also the time when it is last seen. This test is so simple it may be applied by any intelligent person.

Rules for Care of the Colon

The following rules have been tested for years at the Battle Creek Sanitarium and have been found to be efficient, although there are occasionally found cases in which the causes of the constipation are mechanical and require surgical relief: —

1. Intestinal inactivity, or constipation, results in autointoxication, and is one of the most active of all causes of chronic disease. Every chronic invalid should take special care to secure frequent and regular action of the bowels, at least three full movements daily.

2. An effort should be made to move the bowels soon after breakfast, whether or not there is a "call" for bowel movement, and at any other time when even a slight "call" is experienced. A persevering effort should be made to secure three movements daily and at regular times.

3. Cellulose (the indigestible part of vegetable food) is the only element which can increase the bulk of the feces. One to two ounces of cellulose are needed daily. Bran and agaragar are good forms of cellulose.

4. Normally, the bowels move after each meal, and sometimes just after rising. The largest movement generally occurs soon after breakfast.

5. Many persons are suffering from constipation who are not aware of the fact. There are several forms of constipation: (a) *simple constipation*, in which the bowels are only somewhat sluggish or irregular in action; (b) *cumulative or rectal constipation*, in which normal movement of the bowels is prevented by accumulation of masses of feces in the "rectum" or "pelvic" colon; and (c) *latent constipation*, in which the bowels move daily but without complete evacuation of the colon, especially of the lower colon which always occurs in normal defecation. Not infrequently, the symptoms peculiar to latent and cumulative constipation are found present together. It is highly important in every case of constipation that such examinations shall be made as will determine the cause of the constipation. It is only by the aid of such examinations that it becomes possible to make a successful application of curative means.

6. Meals must be regular in time and amount of food taken. Food is the physiologic laxative. A scanty meal or the omission of a meal usually results in the interruption of the intestinal rhythm, — omission of a movement, or an incomplete movement.

7. Fasting, a scanty diet (less than 1600 calories) a liquid diet (milk, gruels, porridges), a diet chiefly consisting of such foods as potatoes, rice, meat, eggs, tea, coffee and condiments, are constipating.

8. Green vegetables (excepting the potato) contain much cellulose, especially the beet root, turnip, parsnip, spinach, cabbage, brussels sprouts, and lettuce; these foods are laxative.

9. Whole grain preparations are rich in cellulose. Scotch brose (oatmeal cooked six minutes) is an excellent laxative food.

10. Half the bulk of dried feces consists of food residues, the other half of germs and of poisonous matter excreted by the intestines, which should be gotten rid of as soon as possible. This is especially important in cases of colitis, since the intestinal mucous membrane is diseased, and in all cases of chronic disease, particularly in cases of autointoxication, Bright's disease, arteriosclerosis, disease of the liver, skin, thyroid gland, heart, and lungs.

11. Exercise promotes bowel action, especially walking, horseback riding, gymnasium exercises, and such exercises as trunk bending, leg raising and deep breathing. Exercises and deep breathing movements taken on the inclined table are especially helpful, and should be practiced systematically and two or three times daily.

12. The cold morning bath often aids bowel action. Various other means are highly beneficial, such as massage of the colon, vibration and kneading of the abdomen, and special exercises of the abdominal muscles. In special cas-

es, application of electricity to the abdominal muscles, also to the rectum and the pelvic colon should be made.

13. In cases in which the abdominal muscles are relaxed, and the colon and other portions of the intestine are prolapsed, an efficient abdominal supporter should be worn either permanently or until the abdominal muscles have become strong enough to hold the viscera in position.

14. Drugs of all sorts must be avoided. They do not cure, and do much harm when repeatedly used. There is no such thing as a harmless laxative drug. Mineral waters and saline laxatives as well as other drugs are harmful, and produce enteritis and colitis sooner or later. They congest the mucous membrane and thus lead to autointoxication.

15. Agar-agar and paraffin are natural and harmless and may be regarded as supplementary foods. They are not digestible and have no influence upon digestion, except to encourage bowel action.

16. Agar-agar (cellulose) aids bowel action by preventing drying and supplying bulk. It also absorbs and carries off toxins. Paraffin lubricates the colon, protects the diseased mucous membrane and hinders absorption of poisons and dissolves and carries off the toxins of putrefaction. These are harmless substances, which may be used continuously without injury, and by regular use render possible the training of the bowels to normal action.

17. In cases in which the measures above indicated do not secure prompt relief from constipation, an X-ray examination by aid of the bismuth meal should be made. By this means, a minute inspection of every part of the intestine is possible. In many cases "kinks," folds, contractions, adhesions, displacements, and other impediments to normal bowel action are found, which may be corrected by application of special measures. Such an examination should be made in all cases of obstinate constipation.

18. The squatting position, secured by using a raised foot-rest in front of the closet seat is a great aid to bowel movement, especially in cases in which the abdominal muscles are relaxed, a condition most common in chronic constipation.

19. If the bowels do not move *three times a day* constipation exists. The constipation may be latent. It is necessary not only that the bowels should move, but that the colon should be completely emptied. A simple test which any one may employ is this: After a bowel movement, take a warm enema, using about three pints of water. About five minutes should be occupied in filling the colon. Note the quantity and character of the evacuation which follows. Often a surprisingly large amount of black, very foul-smelling material will be brought down from an enlarged or pouched caecum where it has been retained perhaps for days. Such accumulations are an exceedingly common cause of headaches, "biliousness," coated tongue, loss of appetite, and other toxic symptoms.

Do not forget that normal bowel action is at least three full evacuations daily.

Food wastes should never be retained more than twenty-five or twenty-six hours at the longest and the normal period is probably sixteen hours or less.

Constipation is one of the greatest causes of disease, misery, inefficiency and premature senility, and should be most earnestly combated. By a persevering effort and the application of known and well tested measures, *every case of constipation may be relieved.*

The Intestinal Flora— When and Why It Must Be Changed

Pasteur discovered that the intestinal tract is swarming with bacteria. Strassburger and other more recent investigators have estimated the number of these organisms produced in the intestinal tract daily to be not less than 150,000,000,000,000, and doubtless the number is sometimes much greater. Pasteur believed and taught that these countless millions of minute organisms were useful and even necessary to the maintenance of the body in health, that they rendered valuable and essential assistance in the process of digestion. More recent studies, however, have shown that Pasteur was in error.

Levin, in the study of Arctic animals at Spitzbergen, showed that more than 50 per cent of the animals in that region have no bacteria in the intestinal tract. Nuttall and Thierfelder showed that guinea pigs brought into the world by Caesarian section may be made to grow without contact with bacteria. Cohendy has quite recently shown that chickens hatched from eggs free from bacteria may be raised and made to thrive on food and drink in an atmosphere entirely free from germs. It is now clearly established that we do not live by the aid of the germs that throng our intestines and swarm upon the surface of the body, but rather that we live in spite of these microbic enemies.

Two Classes — Fermentation Germs and Putrefaction Germs

The germs that are ordinarily found in the human intestine may be divided into two classes; namely, fermentation germs and putrefaction germs. Fermentation germs feed upon carbohydrates; that is, starch, sugar and dextrin; while putrefaction germs feed upon protein — such substances as the white of eggs, the lean of meat, and the curd of milk. Roughly speaking, we may say that fermentation germs feed upon vegetable and putrefaction germs upon animal substances.

These two classes of germs differ very widely in their characteristics and their relation to the human body is in each case based upon the substances which they produce by their activity. Fermentation germs produce for the most part acids, especially lactic and acetic acids, which, in the small quanti-

70

ties in which they are produced in the body, are practically harmless. Putre-faction germs, on the other hand, produce by the decomposition of proteins, especially when acting upon animal proteins, highly poisonous toxins, many of which closely resemble the venom of snakes and minute quantities of which are capable of producing the most alarming and distressing symptoms.

Poisoning from Putrefying Colon Contents

A good illustration of the ill effects of minute doses of these poisons is found in the unpleasant symptoms experienced by contact with putrescible substances, for example, the odors arising from a dead rat in a closet or under the floor, although greatly diluted with air, may give rise to headache, loss of appetite, nausea, and other unpleasant effects. The sickening effects of the odors arising from the fecal discharges of a dog or cat, or of a person accustomed to the free use of meat, clearly demonstrate the potency of these subtle poisons. The bowel discharges of a meat-eater, exposed in a closed room, would in an hour or two render the place intolerable, even to a very robust person. The writer has known vigorous young men to be made very ill with violent attacks of headache through a few hours' contact with such material in laboratory work. A moment's consideration will show that such corrupt and putrescent matters must be capable of producing much greater mischief when in the body than after removal from it. If the mere breathing of the greatly diluted volatile poisons arising from such putrescent matter will produce highly unpleasant effects, how much more grave must be the effects when through the retention within the body of these foul substances all of their poisonous contents are absorbed and sucked up into the blood and circulated throughout the body! In other words, when a person through constipation throws off through the lungs, kidneys and skin a large part of the poisonous matters which ought to have been discharged through the bowel, how great must be the mischief done! There is abundant reason for believing that the poisoning of the body, or so-called autointoxication, which results from the absorption of poisons from the intestine, is the chief cause of most chronic diseases and of premature senility and decay, as well as a very potent and predisposing cause of many acute maladies.

Protective Germs

Normal human beings are born into the world entirely free from bacteria. Not a single germ is found in the interior of the new-born infant. Within a few hours after birth (four to six hours in summer, and twenty hours in winter) the intestines of the infant are found to be swarming with bacteria, the study of which, by Tissier, Escherich and numerous other investigators has shown to be of the harmless sort — namely, the fermentation germs, or acid-formers. It is the presence of these germs that gives to the stools of a healthy young infant a slightly sour odor. A portion of the bowel discharges of the young infant added to milk does not cause putrefaction of the milk, but simply souring or fermentation. These acid-forming germs play a protective role. Thanks to their presence in the intestine, the putrefaction germs cannot thrive, for these organisms cannot grow in the presence of acids. An alkaline medium is needed to promote their growth. Hence, so long as acid-forming germs keep possession of its intestine the infant is safe from the destructive effects of the putrefaction germs, or poison-formers, which are the cause of diarrhea and most other infant troubles. When by the use of cow's milk (that is, ordinary commercial milk), or by other errors in feeding, such as the giving of meat or fish, overwhelming numbers of putrefaction germs are introduced into the intestine and the infant's stools become dark-colored and bad-smelling, then the experienced mother or nurse, as well as the doctor, knows that the child, if not already sick, will soon be sick, and the sickness will be due to the poisons produced by these enemies of life, the germs of putrefaction.

As the child advances in years the putrefaction germs increase in number in the intestine. Through the use of meat, highly active putrefaction germs are introduced into the intestine and grow and multiply in great numbers, so that the stools become very offensive and chronic autointoxication results. The ultimate effects are constipation, colitis, so-called biliousness, gastritis, inflammation of the gall ducts, gall stones, skin diseases of various sorts, neurasthenia, and in later years Bright's disease, hardening of the arteries, high blood-pressure, apoplexy, paralysis, insomnia, mental depression, and even insanity.

The Cause of Old Age

Metchnikoff has clearly shown that these putrefaction germs are the cause of early senility, premature old age and death. Among the worst of the putrefaction germs which are commonly found in the intestine in the diseased conditions of adult life are the *bacillus coli, Welch's bacillus, bacillus proteus, bacillus subtilis, streptococcus, enterococcus, bacillus putrificus, bacillus paracoli,* and sometimes the typhoid bacillus. All of these germs produce most virulent poisons, and when present in the feces in large numbers they are certain proof of the existence of chronic intestinal autointoxication, even though the characteristic symptoms of autointoxication have not yet appeared. A coated tongue, a sallow complexion, dark circles around the eyes, appearance of brown spots upon the hands or other parts (the so-called liver spots), offensive breath and perspiration, the discharge of foul-smelling gases from the bowels, putrid stools, a thin, inelastic, parchment-like skin, dullness of mind, inability to concentrate the mind, mental irritability or depression without cause, cold hands and feet, perspiration of the hands and feet, chronic headache, attacks of migraine or sick headache — these and a score of other symptoms which might be mentioned are certain indications of chronic poisoning, prompt attention to which may prevent the development of later more serious conditions, such as hardening of the arteries, Bright's disease, with albumen and casts in the urine, or apoplexy with paralysis. Grave symptoms of autointoxication do not appear until after the mechanism of the body, through which nature deals with poisons, destroying and eliminating them, has broken down and failed to accomplish its purpose as a result of the overwhelming amount of work which has been thrown upon it. Hence, the appearance of symptoms of autointoxication indicates that the body has already become crippled and that the matter must receive serious and immediate attention.

Reforming the Intestinal Flora

Eminent progressive medical men the world over are rapidly coming to recognize that changing the intestinal flora is an important factor in the treatment of all forms of chronic disease and that in the great majority of chronic diseases it is the one essential thing. Modern researches have clearly shown that the great benefit that has been known to be derived from those methods of treatment which have been most successful have really been due to the influence of these measures upon the intestinal flora.

We may mention, for example, the temporary benefit derived by the tens of thousands of persons who annually visit mineral springs, the waters of which possess laxative properties. Such resorts are popular in all parts of the world, and the benefit derived from the use of their waters is sufficient to attract countless multitudes of visitors year after year; but that these patients are never cured, no matter how much temporary benefit they may derive from the thorough emptying of their intestines and the unloading of accumulated poisons, is shown by the fact that they always return, often being compelled to return at increasingly frequent intervals, the effect of mineral water as well as of other laxatives being to produce colitis, or infection of the colon thus in the end doing great harm.

Results or Changing the Flora

Again, we find in the remarkable effects which have been obtained by various special dietaries an equally good illustration of the curative value of means which influence the intestinal flora. The grape cure, the apple, peach, cherry and other fruit cures, the milk, buttermilk and whey cures — all of these cures operate through their influence upon the intestinal flora. The same statement may also apply to the raw food cure, which acquired considerable vogue some years ago.

Fruits and milk are substances which ferment but do not putrefy. Hence, when the diet is exclusively confined to these articles, fermentative changes rather than putrefaction take place in the intestine, acids are formed instead of poisons, and for the time being the body is delivered from the destructive influence of the highly potent toxins produced by putrefactive germs when active either within the body or outside of it. Raw foods of a vegetable character are alive and hence able to resist the action of bacteria. Vegetable foods taken in raw or uncooked state are digested before it is possible for them to undergo destructive changes, and thus their use discourages the growth of bacteria in the intestine, especially those of the putrefactive sort. There are also other benefits from the use of uncooked food.

Dangerous Germs Made Harmless

Bienstock showed that the colon germs, which, in the presence of protein (meat, eggs, etc.), produce indol and other highly active poisons capable of causing hardening of the arteries, headache, probably Bright's disease, and numerous other disorders, are, in the presence of sugar, incapable of producing these poisonous substances, producing instead harmless acids.

Sir Lauder Brunton, of England, and more recently Kennan, in this country, have shown that this is true of practically all putrefactive germs; that is, the germs which cause putrefaction when growing on protein will, if supplied with a sufficient amount of sugar, cease to produce putrefactive poisons and produce fermentation with harmless acids instead. In other words, putrefaction germs may be reformed by simply feeding them with sugar. This explains the fact that eggs, which of all substances most readily undergo putrefaction, may be perfectly preserved by the addition of sugar. It also explains the fact that the pioneer housewife and the nomadic Arab are able to maintain a supply of fresh meat by immersing cutlets in cow's milk or camel's milk. The writer has in his possession a beefsteak which has been kept in a state of perfect preservation for twelve years (since June, 1906), by immersion in buttermilk made from a culture of the *Bacillus Bulgaricus* (the buttermilk has been changed frequently).

It appears, then, that putrefactive organisms, which are now recognized as among the most common and deadly enemies of human life, may actually become harmless and even useful by supplying them with sugar, provided this can be done at the proper time and in the proper place. The proportion of sugar must be at least two per cent.

How to Change the Intestinal Flora

After studying this question for more than twenty years, or ever since the appearance of Bouchard's great work, "Autointoxication in Disease, or Self-Poisoning of the Individual," the writer became fully persuaded that it is possible to change the intestinal flora, and that this change is one of the most practical and most important means of combating the great majority of the chronic diseases with which the physician has to deal. A method which has been thoroughly tested may be briefly described as follows:

To change the intestinal flora, three things are essential:

1. To so regulate the diet that there will be left in the colon no putrescible food residues. This is accomplished by eliminating from the diet for a few days all animal proteins, that is, meat, milk, and eggs, and also vegetable foods rich in protein, such as beans, peas, and cereals. Fats are also excluded because they delay the movement of the food through the stomach and small intestine and encourage putrefaction in the colon. A diet consisting wholly of fruits or fruits and fresh green vegetables such as lettuce or cabbage, celery, and other green things is best. Malt sugar or milk sugar may be used freely.

2. The activity of the bowels must be increased to such a degree that the food residues will not be retained in the colon long enough to undergo putrefaction. This requires three or four efficient bowel movements daily, or at least one bowel movement after each meal. By the free use of bran or agar-agar and paraffin oil in some form, spontaneous movements may usually be secured. When necessary, the colon may be emptied by a thorough enema once or twice a day, using water at a temperature of 80°F. or warm water (100°F.), followed by cool water.

In children and in some persons who enjoy superb health, the bowels move four times daily; before breakfast, after breakfast, after dinner, and at bedtime.

The idea entertained by many persons that frequent bowel movement is weakening, is wholly erroneous. The bowels move often in cases of diarrhoea for the purpose of carrying away poisons produced in the intestine by invading germs. The weakness felt is not due to the bowel movements but to the poisons, some portion of which is absorbed in spite of Nature's vigorous efforts to eliminate them.

3. A third factor of importance, though less essential than the preceding, is the introduction of protective organisms, the lactic acid forming ferments or so-called buttermilk germs. There are several of these, and they are more effective in combination than alone. These ferments are best used at first in whey cultures rather than in milk, and large amounts of milk sugar (6 to 8 ounces daily) should be used with them. In extreme cases and when rapid results are desired, the cultures should be used by enema, as well as by mouth, thus planting the protective germs where they are most needed and may render most effective service.

"The Fruit Regimen"

The combination of these methods constitutes the "Fruit Regimen," a few days of which rarely fails to clear the tongue, sweeten the breath, and dissipate the foul odor of the stools, which become odorless or acquire a slight sour odor.

When the tongue has been cleared, the "Milk Regimen" may be utilized with great advantage as a means of fixing in the intestine the protective germs which the "Fruit Regimen" has introduced.

The "Milk Regimen" is much the same as the "Fruit Regimen" except that milk is substituted for fruit and is given every half hour and to the extent of five or six quarts daily. On this regimen, the bowels should move very freely, and the stools should be much like those of an infant.

After two or three weeks of the "Milk Regimen," the patient is prepared for the Antitoxic Diet or Regimen.

Antitoxic Diet

This diet consists chiefly of fruits, cereals, and fresh vegetables, and should include a considerable amount of uncooked vegetables, such as lettuce, cucumbers and cabbage. The experiments at the Pasteur Institute have shown that potatoes and dates are particularly valuable as antitoxic foods, probably because the carbohydrates which they contain — starch in the potato, and sugar in the date — are not fully absorbed in the small intestine and reach the colon in larger amount than do the carbohydrates of most other foods. Carrots also were shown by Metchnikoff s experiments to be a valuable antitoxic food. Another specially valuable food, of which the writer has made much use with excellent success is oatmeal prepared by short cooking. The steel-cut oats or old-fashioned Scotch oats are better for the purpose than rolled oats. Instead of cooking a long time so as to insure the complete conversion of all the starch, the oatmeal should be stirred into boiling water and cooked for five minutes, then set aside for five minutes more, and then served. Oats prepared in this way constitute the brose of the Scotch Highlanders, and is most palatable. Nevertheless, a considerable portion is imperfectly cooked and hence is not readily acted upon by the saliva and intestinal juices, and thus finds its way into the colon, where it may feed the fermentation germs and by its presence prevent the putrefaction germs from making poisons by the decomposition of protein. This protective action may be increased by the addition of wheat bran to the oatmeal in the proportion of one part to three by volume measure. The bran will hasten the passage of the oatmeal through the intestinal canal and will thus increase the amount of carbohydrate which reaches the colon.

An excellent breakfast food consists of equal parts by measure of corn meal, steel-cut oats and sterilized bran, cooked six to ten minutes.

The free use of such saccharine fruits as prunes, figs, and raisins is also a valuable means of introducing carbohydrates in the most available form, since the germs which live in the colon thrive better on a diet of sugar than any other form of carbohydrates. Purple figs soaked in cold water for twenty-four hours are a very palatable laxative food.

The Colon Not Intended to be a Sewer

Nature never intended that the interior of the human intestine should be degraded to the condition of a privy vault or an obstructed sewer, flooding the blood with brain-and-nerve-paralyzing and disease-breeding poisons. This is clearly evident, not only by the observations of Levin at Spitzbergen, above referred to, but also by the discovery in South America of a parrot which lives wholly upon bananas, and the fecal discharges of which have the fragrance of bananas and are inoffensive as bananas themselves. What natural reason can be shown that food that enters the body clean, sweet and sterile should leave the body in a state horribly loathsome with corruption?

Clean blood is a first essential for health of body and mind. Clean blood is impossible without a clean colon. Constipation is a fundamental and almost universal evil which is the root of more human ills and perhaps more human misery, moral and mental as well as physical than any other cause. Fortunately it is not an incurable condition. The average civilized colon is badly crippled, but it may be greatly helped. An intelligent application of up-to-date knowledge of colon conditions may attain success in the most discouraging cases.

Every case of constipation is curable, but not by means of any panacea. Each case must be studied and individual conditions must be dealt with in an intelligent and rational manner.

The successful treatment of chronic constipation requires a careful study of each individual case in the light of modern knowledge of the physiology of the colon and in obstinate cases the whole alimentary canal must be inspected by means of the X-ray with the opaque meal and enema.

The intestinal flora must be changed. This is absolutely necessary to conquer constipation. Putrefactive poisons paralyze the colon, while the harmless acids of fermentation are the normal stimulants of the intestine, hence the necessity for exchanging the wild bacteria for the protective germs which nature provides as a bulwark against disease.

The details of methods of treatment, diet, how to change the intestinal flora, and other matters that pertain to the practical management of the colon is given in other works by the author, especially "Colon Hygiene," and "Autointoxication."

By the use of these methods, many persons thought to be proper subjects for surgical treatment may be wholly relieved and restored to comfort and usefulness. The suffering of subjects of chronic autointoxication is often so great that they are quite willing to submit to any treatment, medical or surgical, no matter how drastic, provided only that a fair prospect of relief is held out to them.

With high hopes of relief from chronic miseries, hundreds of persons have undergone operations for removal of the appendix, "short-circuiting," or even removal of the colon, or some other radical procedure, and have then found themselves subject to the same miseries as before, often with aggravated intensity.

The truth is that the "kinks," and most other morbid conditions which are thought to require surgical interference, are results rather than causes of the fundamental mischiefs, which must be corrected before any permanent benefit will be secured.

The notion that the appendix is a useless "relic" and the colon a handicap and a menace which should have been long ago left behind in the march of evolution, is not in harmony with sound scientific principles. Nature is wise. Because the purpose of an organ is not understood, we should not feel at liberty to denounce it as cumbersome and dangerous. It is but a few years since the spleen was looked upon as a superfluous organ, if not a burden to the bodily economy. Now, we know that the functions of the spleen are of highest importance to the body. While it is possible for a person to live without it, at least for several years, its activity is known to be essential to the perfect working of the bodily machinery, especially of the defensive mechanisms.

The thyroid gland was for ages regarded as of no use to an adult, though regarded of use in the early periods of development before birth and during the first months of infancy. Now, we know that this gland has most important duties to perform in connection with nutrition, especially in the protection of the body against the poisons produced in the colon by the putrefaction of protein. Dogs whose thyroids have been removed die when fed on meat, but thrive on a diet from which meat is excluded, such as bread and milk.

A minute body in the brain, not larger than a pea, once a mere anatomical curiosity, thought by the philosopher, Descartes, to be the seat of the soul, is now known to play a very important part in regulating growth. Disease of this minute structure may be accompanied by loss of bodily symmetry. The hands and feet become gigantic in size, all out of proportion to the rest of the body. The nose or the lower jaw may become immensely too large for the rest of the face.

The appendix vermiformis, long regarded as a vestige and a trouble maker, is now known to be a leading factor in the highly important lubricating system of the colon. It is a great mucous follicle and pours out its lubricating mucus at just the point where it is most needed. Prof. MacEwen, of Edinburgh, an eminent Scotch surgeon, and also the late Prof. Andrews, a distinguished Chicago surgeon, called attention to this useful function of the appendix many years ago. A person who has had his appendix removed, has lost a valuable part of his lubricating mechanism.

Such persons generally find it necessary to make constant use of paraffin oil to replace the function of the lost organ.

As a matter of fact, a very large proportion of the appendices which are removed have no direct connection with the complaints for relief from which the operation is performed. After the operation, the patient suffers the same as before.

The same things may be said of the colon. It is not a useless organ. Its purpose is to secure regular and rhythmical discharge of the food residues and body wastes instead of a constant discharge as in some birds and fishes, in which the colon is so short as to be of little use as a reservoir. When the colon is removed, nature proceeds to make a new reservoir by dilating the lower end of the ileum until it becomes as large as the normal colon.

It has become evident that the fault with the modern colon is not that it is superfluous, but that it has been systematically abused by requiring it to deal with material which it was never intended to handle, as pointed out by the eminent Professor Keith of London. Nature intended the colon of man, as those of other primates, the orang and the chimpanzee, to be used as a reservoir for holding for a few hours the residues of fruits and roots and tender shoots, the indigestible seeds, skins, and fibres of vegetable food stuffs, material incapable of undergoing putrefaction or giving rise to poisonous products of any sort. But by becoming a meat eater man has compelled his colon to deal with the putrescent fragments of undigested flesh, highly offensive material which the short colons of carnivorous animals dismiss quickly and handle with little injury, but which stored up in the capacious human colon for many hours, even several days, become a seething mass of corruption, a veritable Pandora's box of disease.

And so the conclusion to which sound reason and experience lead us is that the colon does not need to be eliminated by evolution or removed by surgery (except when hopelessly diseased), but that it needs to be reformed by proper training and return to a natural dietary. That these measures are successful has been demonstrated by the experience of the Battle Creek Sanitarium where they have been systematically employed in the treatment of more than one hundred thousand invalids within the last forty years, most of whom were suffering from chronic constipation and its consequences.

Nuts - A Coming Food Staple

In these days when the question of foodstuffs is daily becoming more urgent and absorbing it is natural that all available sources of supplies to meet one of the most urgent of all our human needs should be made the subject of careful investigation. The exigencies of the great European war have compelled not only Germany but others of the belligerent nations to study nutritive values and the economics of food more critically than ever before. Every possible source of food supply is being drawn upon to the fullest extent possible by the nations of Central Europe. Efforts have been made to extract nutrient material from such unpromising sources as straw and sawdust, naturally with no encouraging measure of success.

The writer has followed these researches and discussions with great interest. Numerous important facts in relation to human nutrition which have been long known to scientists but of which the common people have been ignorant have been brought to the attention of the hungry masses and have received practical application in the masterly efforts which have been made for their relief. It is probable that the problem of human nutrition is at the present time being solved in a more scientific and practical way by the German people than the world has ever seen done before.

In all this discussion, however, one of the first and most striking facts upon which public attention was focused after the beginning of the great conflict was the necessity for limiting the supply of flesh foods. The reason for this is obvious. All the densely populated nations of Europe depend chiefly upon outside sources for their meat supplies. This must be true of any densely populated country for the reason that an acre of land that is devoted to wheat, for example, will produce nearly ten times as much protein, one of the most essential of all the food principles, as the same area of land devoted to pasturage for beef cattle and, as will be shown later in this paper, the same land devoted to nuts may produce an even greater amount of food protein together with other essential food principles. Notwithstanding this fact, the writer has seen no mention made of nuts in the discussions of food supplies which have grown out of the European war. The explanation doubtless is to be found in the fact that nuts have heretofore cut so small a figure in national food supplies that, under the present emergency conditions, they are naturally overlooked entirely.

As a matter of fact, nuts have been used as a luxury rather than as a staple article of food; but as the public become better informed respecting the high food value of nuts and especially in view of the steadily rising cost of flesh meats, the nut is certain to gain higher appreciation, and the writer has no doubt that sometime in the future nuts will become a leading constituent of the national bill of fare and in so doing, will displace certain foodstuffs which today are held in high esteem but which in the broader light of the next century will be regarded as objectionable and inferior foods and will give place to the products of the various varieties of nut trees which will then be recognized as the choicest of all foods.

Botanically, a nut is a fruit; but nuts differ so widely both in composition and appearance from the foods commonly called fruits that they are properly classed by themselves. In nutritive value the nut far exceeds all other food substances; for example, the average number of food units per pound furnished by half a dozen of the more common varieties of nuts is 3231 calories while the average of the same number of varieties of cereals is 1654 calories, half the value of nuts. The average food value of the best vegetables is 300 calories per pound and of the best fresh fruits grown in this country is 278 calories. The average value of the six principal flesh foods is 810 calories per pound or one-fourth that of nuts.

The superior nutritive value of nuts is clearly shown by the following tables based upon the analyses of Atwater and others:

Composition and Fuel Value of the Edible Portion of Nuts.

	Protein	Fats	Carbohy-drates	Ash	Food value per pound
	per ct.	per ct.	per ct.	per ct.	Calories
Almonds 21.0	54.9	17.3	2.0	3,030
Brazil nuts 17.0	66.8	7.0	3.9	3,329
Filberts 15.6	65.3	13.0	2.4	3,432
Hickory nuts 15.4	67.4	11.4	2.1	3,495
Pecan nuts 11.0	71.2	13.3	1.5	3,633
English walnuts ...16.7	64.4	14.8	1.3	3,305
Chestnuts, fresh ... 6.2	5.4	42.1	1.3	1,125
Chestnuts, dried ...10.7	7.0	74.2	2.2	1,875
Acorns 8.1	37.4	48.0	2.4	2,718
Beechnuts 21.9	57.4	13.2	3.5	3,263
Butternuts 27.9	61.2	3.4	3.0	3,371
Black walnuts 27.6	56.3	11.7	1.9	3,105
Cocoanuts 5.7	50.6	27.9	1.7	2,986
Cocoanuts shredded . 6.3	57.3	31.6	1.3	3,125
Pistachios, kernels..22.6	54.5	15.6	3.1	3,010
Pine nuts or pinons 14.6	61.9	17.3	2.8	3,364
Peanuts, raw 25.8	38.6	24.4	2.0	2,560
Peanuts, roasted ...30.5	49.2	16.2	2.5	3,177
Litchi nuts 2.9	.2	77.5	1.5	1,453

With the exception of smoked bacon, there is no flesh food which even approaches the nut in nutritive value, and bacon owes its high value to the fact that it consists almost exclusively of fat.

That the nut is appreciated as a dainty is attested by the frequency with which it appears as a dessert and the extensive use of various nuts as confections. That nuts do not hold a more prominent place in the national bill of fare is due chiefly to two causes; first, the popular idea that nuts are highly indigestible, and second, their comparatively high price.

The notion that nuts are difficult of digestion has really no foundation in fact. The idea is probably the natural outgrowth of the custom of eating nuts at the close of a meal when an abundance, more likely a super-abundance, of highly nutritious foods has already been eaten and the equally injurious custom of eating nuts between meals. Neglect of thorough mastication must also be mentioned as a common cause of indigestion following the use of nuts. Nuts are generally eaten dry and have a firm hard flesh which requires thorough use of the organs of mastication to prepare them for the action of the several digestive juices. Experiments made in Germany showed that nuts are not digested at all but pass through the alimentary canal like foreign bodies unless reduced to a smooth paste in the mouth. Particles of nuts the size of small seeds wholly escaped digestion.

The Origin of Peanut Butter

Having been for more than fifty years actively interested in promoting the use of nuts as a staple food, I have given considerable thought and study to their dietetic value and have made many experiments. About twenty-five years ago it occurred to me that one of the above objections to the extensive dietetic use of nuts might be overcome by mechanical preparation of the nut before serving so as to reduce it to a smooth paste and thus insure the preparation for digestion which the average eater is prone to neglect. The result was a product which I called peanut butter. I was much surprised at the readiness with which the product sprang into public favor. Several years ago I was informed by a wholesale grocer of Chicago that the firm's sales of peanut butter amounted on an average to a carload a week. I think it is safe to estimate that not less than one thousand carloads of this product are annually consumed in this country. The increased demand for peanuts for making peanut butter led to the development of "corners" in the peanut market and doubled the price and the annual production.

I am citing my experience with the peanut not for the purpose of recommending this product, for I am obliged to confess that I was soon compelled to abandon the use of peanut butter prepared from roasted nuts, for the reason that the process of roasting renders the nut indigestible to such a degree that it was not adapted to the use of invalids, but simply as an illustration of the readiness with which the public accepts a new dietetic idea when it happens to strike the popular fancy.

Delicious nut butters may be prepared from true nuts such as the almond, filbert, and pine nut, by blanching and crushing, without roasting. Peanuts require steam roasting.

Ways must be found to render the use of nuts practical by adapting them to our culinary and dietetic customs and to overcome the popular objection to their use by a widespread and efficient campaign of education.

Food Economy

It has long been predicted by economists that the time would come when a densely populated world would be compelled to derive its sustenance directly from the soil. The present high prices of meat were anticipated more than twenty years ago by the officials of the United States Department of Agriculture. The increase of our human population and the decrease of our animal population have both progressed more rapidly than was anticipated, and the artificial conditions imposed by the world war have still further increased the price of meat and made meatless days a necessity. Thus the question, Is meat essential to complete human nutrition? has become most pertinent.

A fundamental error is embodied in the popular faith in the high protein ration. The physiologists are at least partly at fault. Liebig's dictum, which made protein the essential food factor in supporting work, has misled the whole civilized world for more than half a century. The dietaries of institutions, armies, whole nations have been based upon a conception which modern science has shown to be utterly false, and the result has been an economic loss which staggers belief, and a destruction of human life and efficiency which overshadows most other malign influences.

As an abstract scientific proposition this question was answered by the physiologists years ago by laboratory experiments. According to Magnus

Levy, one of the world's most eminent authorities, "It is indeed true that the vegetable albuminous substances as they occur in nature are equal in nutritive value to an equivalent protein of animal origin."

More recent studies, however, by McCollum and others have shown that the selection of the vegetable foodstuffs which shall compose the bill-of-fare is not a matter of indifference. There is a difference in proteins. Every vegetable produces proteins which are peculiar to itself. Animal proteins also differ, but apparently less widely than do vegetable proteins, and many vegetable proteins differ very greatly in character from those which compose the highly vitalized parts of the human body.

Fortunately, vegetable proteins do not all differ in the same way. Some differ in one direction, others in the exact opposite direction. And so by the proper selection of vegetable foodstuffs it is possible to make a combination which will supply the human body with just the sort of material which it requires for building purposes and for repairs.

Taking the protein of the human body for a standard, it is found that the proteins which are found in cereals, green and root vegetables, legumes and most other vegetable products are incomplete. They are lacking in certain elements which are absolutely essential to the building of healthy human blood and tissues.

Careful chemical analysis, however, has shown in recent years that the proteins of nuts, or at least of some of them, are complete proteins. Nuts, in fact, furnish proteins of such fine quality that they are capable of complementing other foodstuffs. Their proteins supply the elements necessary to render complete the proteins of cereals and other vegetable foods. This discovery is one of the highest importance since it opens a door of escape for the race from the threatened extinction by starvation at some future period, perhaps not so very remote.

Advantages of a Nut Diet

This fact places the nut in an exceedingly important position as a foodstuff. In face of vanishing meat supplies it is most comforting to know that meats of all sorts may be safely replaced by nuts not only without loss, but with a decided gain. Nuts have several advantages over flesh foods which are well worth considering.

1. Nuts are free from waste products, uric acid, urea, carnine, and other tissue wastes.

2. Nuts are aseptic, free from putrefactive bacteria, and do not readily undergo decay either in the body or outside of it. Meats, on the other hand, are practically always in an advanced stage of putrefaction, as found in the meat markets. Ordinary meats contain from three million to ten times that number of bacteria per ounce, and such meats as Hamburger steak often contain more than a billion putrefactive organisms to the ounce. Nuts are clean and sweet.

3. Nuts are free from trichinae, tapeworm, and other parasites, as well as other infections due to specific disease. Nuts are in good health when gathered and remain so until eaten. The contrast between the delectable product of the beautiful walnut, chestnut or pecan tree and the abbatoir recalls the story of the Tennessee school teacher who was told when she made inquiry about a certain shoulder of pork which had been promised in part payment for services but had not arrived, "Dad didn't kill the pig;" "and why not," said the teacher. "Because," replied the observing youngster, "He got well." Nearly all the cows slaughtered are tuberculous. They are killed to be eaten because too sick to longer serve as community wet nurses.

It is also worthy of note that the fat of nuts exists in a finely divided state and that in the chewing of nuts a fine emulsion is produced so that nuts enter the stomach in a form best adapted for prompt digestion.

Another question which will naturally arise is this: if nuts are to be granted the place of a staple in our list of food supplies, will it be safe to accept them as a substitute for flesh foods?

Beefsteak with many people has become a veritable fetish, but the experiments of Chittenden and others have demonstrated that the amount of protein needed by the body daily is so small that it is scarcely possible to arrange a bill of fare to include flesh foods without making the protein intake excessive. This is because the ordinary foodstuffs other than meat contain a sufficient amount of protein to meet the needs of the body. Nuts present their protein in combination with so large a proportion of easily digestible fat that there is comparatively little danger of getting an excess.

It is also worthy of note that the protein of nuts is superior in quality to that of ordinary vegetables or meats. The careful analyses made in recent years have shown that the protein of nuts, at least of a number of them, contain all the elements needed for building up complete body proteins; in other words, nuts furnish perfect proteins, which are not supplied so abundantly by any other vegetable product.

A False Economy

From an economic standpoint, the rearing of animals for food is a monstrous extravagance. According to Professor Henry, dean of the Agricultural Department of the University of Wisconsin, and author of an authoritative work on foods and feeding, one hundred pounds of food fed to a steer produce less than three pounds of food in the form of flesh. In other words, we must feed the steer thirty-three pounds of corn in order to get back one pound of food in the form of steak. Such an extravagant waste can be tolerated only so long as it is possible to produce a large excess of foodstuffs. It is stated, as a matter of fact, that at the present time scarcely more than ten per cent, of the corn raised in the United States is directly consumed by human beings. A large part of it is wasted in feeding to animals. This economic loss has been long known to practical men but it has been regarded as unavoidable since meat has been supposed to be absolutely essential as an article of food; but the experience of Germany since the beginning of the present war, as well as of Japan, China, and India for many centuries, has fully demonstrated the possibility of eliminating meat from the national bill of fare.

The use of nuts as a staple article of food is not an experiment. All the higher apes, man's nearest relatives in the animal world, thrive on nuts. Many savage tribes live very largely on nuts. The Indians of the foothills of California gather every fall large quantities of nuts which they store for winter use. The early settlers of California reported that many tribes of Indians in that part of the United States lived almost wholly upon acorns. Before the great oak forests of this country were cut down, many millions of hogs were fattened on mast, and the price of pork depended more upon the acorn crop than on the corn crop. The peasantry of southern France and northern Italy during half the year make two meals a day on chestnuts.

As a matter of fact, milk and eggs supply essentially the same protein that is furnished by meat, and milk protein in some respects superior to that of meat; but milk is rapidly rising in price and will doubtless go still higher for the reason that for every pound of food in the form of milk it is necessary to feed a cow more than five times the amount of food obtained; and for every pound of food in the form of eggs we must throw away nearly twenty pounds of good food. So it is more than probable that the time may not be far distant when the people of this country, like those of some other countries, and like our primitive ancestors who lived wholly upon the products of the forests, and our modern biological relatives, the orang-utan, the chimpanzee, and the gorilla, must depend chiefly upon the products of the vegetable kingdom for their sustenance with the addition of eggs and milk.

It is important then to know that, if such a time comes, it would be possible so to arrange the bill of fare that the race may lose nothing of vigor or energy because of the restriction in diet. As a matter of fact, there is good reason to believe that if man had never acquired his present omnivorous habits and had adhered to his original vegetable regimen, he might have escaped a very large proportion of the multitudinous ills which have greatly impaired his efficiency and are even threatening extinction of the race.

The high price of meat of which so much complaint has been made in recent years is not likely to recede. The high price is not due to manipulations of the market, but to natural causes the chief of which is the limitation of pasturage and is the consequence of a decrease in the number of livestock. As the country becomes more and more densely settled, the difficulty of supplying the demand for meat will increase, and in time the necessity for utilizing every foot of ground in the most efficient manner, will necessarily bring about a change in the dietetic habits of the people. Not one example can be found in the world of a densely populated country dependent upon its own resources in which flesh foods constitute any considerable part of the national bill of fare. Since Germany has been nearly shut off from the outside world by the present war, the government has found it necessary to restrict the consumption of meat to one-half pound per week for each adult. All other European countries are equally dependent on outside sources for their meat supply.

The time will certainly come when nuts and nut trees will become a most important food resource. If a reform in this direction could be effected within the next ten years, the result would be a disappearance to a large extent of the complaint of the high cost of living. James Hill said the basis for complaint was not the high cost of living, but the cost of high living. I should prefer to say that the real cause for complaint was wrong living rather than high living, or necessarily high cost. With right living the cost will be automatically reduced. For example, suppose a person were content to choose the peanut as his chief source of protein and fat, the elimination of the butcher's bill for meat and the grocer's bill for butter would at once cut out two-thirds of the expense incurred for food.

A Personal Experience

When a student in college more than forty years ago, the writer lived three months on a diet such as has been above suggested, at an average expense of exactly six cents a day. This was the total amount expended for raw food-stuffs. I paid my landlady five times as much for preparing and serving the food, and had reason for believing that some portion of my supplies was utilized by others than myself. As evidence of the fact that the experiment was not dangerous, I may add that I have pursued the same meatless dietary during my entire lifetime since, as I had done for ten years before, and in my sixty-seventh am still alive and hard at work.

Man is naturally a frugivorous animal. According to Cuvier, the renowned French naturalist, the natural diet of human beings, like that of those other primates, the orangutan, the chimpanzee, and the gorilla, consists of fruits, nuts, tender shoots and grains.

A sturdy Scotch highlander told me that his diet consisted of brose, bannocks, and potatoes, and that he rarely ever tasted meat. When asked what he fed his dogs, he replied, "The same as I eat myself, sir." The highbred fox-hounds of the southern states are fed on cornmeal, oatmeal and bread, and rarely taste flesh of any sort. Dogs thus fed are hardier, healthier, have more endurance, better wind, keener scent, greater intelligence, and are more easily trained than meat fed dogs. A diet which is safe for carnivorous animals must certainly be safe for human beings who belong to a class of animals all representatives of which, with the exception of man, are flesh abstainers.

Some years ago I experimented with various sorts of carnivorous animals for the purpose of ascertaining whether nuts could be made a complete substitute for meat. Among the various animals utilized for the experiment was a young wolf from the northwest that had never eaten anything but fresh raw meat. After giving the animal one day to get accustomed to its new surroundings and to acquire a good appetite I gave him a breakfast of nuts properly prepared and was delighted to find that he took to the new ration without the slightest hesitation and remained in excellent health during the several months of the experiment. I succeeded perfectly in substituting nuts for meat with all the animals experimented upon including a fish hawk, with the single exception of an ancient bald-headed eagle which refused to be converted.

The First Mammals Were Nut-Eaters

I have long had a suspicion that the so-called carnivorous animals were all at some remote time nut-eaters; the so-called carnivorous teeth would be as useful in tearing off the husks of cocoanuts and similar fruits as for tearing and eating flesh.

It is gratifying to be assured by the Eminent Prof. Matthews, that the first mammals were nut-eaters and vegetarians and that our remote ancestors were nut and fruit eaters. They may have gobbled an insect now and then but their staple food was fruits and nuts with tender shoots and succulent roots, which is still true of those old fashioned forest folks, the primates of which the orang-utan, the chimpanzee and the gorilla are consistent representatives, while their near relatives, also a primate, civilized man, has departed from his original bill of fare and has exploited the bills of fare of the whole animal kingdom.

The keeper of the famous big apes of the London Zoo informed me that they were never given meat. Even the small monkeys, generally regarded as insectivorous, were confined to a rigid vegetarian fare and were thriving.

Whole races of men, comprising many millions, live their entire lives without meats of any sort, and when fed a sufficient amount are wonderfully vigorous, prolific, enduring and intelligent. Witness the Brahmins of India, the Buddhists of China and Japan and the teeming millions of Central Africa.

The World's Pedestrian Record Won by a Nut Eater

Carl Mann, the winner of the great walking match between Berlin and Dresden, performed his great feat on a diet of nuts with lettuce and fruits.

Weston, the long distance champion, never eats meat when on a long walk. The Tarahumara Indians, the fleetest and most enduring runners in the world, are strict vegetarians. The gorilla, the king of the Congo forests, is a nut-feeder. Milo, the mighty Greek, was a flesh-abstainer as was also Pythagoras, the first of the Greek philosophers, Seneca, the noble Roman senator and Plutarch, the famous biographer. The writer has excluded meat from his bill of fare for more than fifty years, and has within the last forty years, supervised the treatment of more than a hundred thousand sick people at the Battle Creek Sanitarium on a meatless diet and superintended the activities of a family of workers averaging for many years more than 1000, who are also flesh-abstainers, no meat being served at the Sanitarium to either patients or workers.

Even carnivorous animals flourish on a diet of nuts with other vegetable foods and cooked cereals. The Turks mix nuts with their pilaff of rice and the Armenians add nuts to their boolghoor, a dish prepared from wheat which has been cooked and dried.

With the addition of milk or eggs, a fleshless diet is not only absolutely safe and sufficient but in every way superior to a flesh diet.

Nuts May Save the Race

In view of these facts it is most interesting to know that in nuts, the most neglected of all well-known food products, we find the assurance of an ample and complete food supply for all future time, even though necessity should compel the total abandonment of our present forms of animal industry.

One of the great advantages of the nut is that with few exceptions, it may be eaten direct from the hand of nature without culinary preparation of any sort. Indeed, the common custom in offering nuts as dessert is an acknowledgment that the refined chemistry of nature's laboratory permits of no improvement by the clumsy methods of the kitchen.

The Nut is a Fruit with a Shell

In the process of ripening, the actinic rays of the sun digest the crude starch found in the green fruit and convert it into delicious fats and sugars ready for prompt utilization. The protein of the nut resembles the casein of milk and requires no cooking to render it readily digestible. The only preparation the nut needs is thorough mastication to insure the prompt admixture and action of the digestive fluids. Mastication is chiefly a mechanical process and may be very largely substituted by crushing the nut into a paste or grinding it into a fine meal.

More than fifty years ago it had been demonstrated that flesh foods are not an essential part of the dietary of man. Cuvier, the great French naturalist had stated that man's natural diet was the same as that of the chimpanzee and the orang-utan and consisted of fruits, nuts, soft grains and tender shoots.

The evidence of the scientific accuracy of Cuvier's statement was so conclusive that the writer adopted the natural diet and has followed it since. This journal, during this time, has very earnestly advocated the biologic diet and thousands of people have been persuaded to adopt it.

In the Battle Greek Sanitarium more than 100,000 sick people besides employees, students, friends of patients and guests, numbering at least half as many more persons have been introduced to a fleshless bill of fare often with very evident and very great benefit.

In this institution no small interest has been taken in nuts as a part of nature's scheme of human feeding, and a conspicuous place has been given them in our bill of fare. During all this period extensive inquiries have been carried on, having for their purpose the development of the nutritive proper-ties of all sorts of foodstuffs and many thousands of experiments with nuts have been made in food laboratories. In the course of these experiments the simple process of making peanut butter was hit upon which has since devel-oped into a great industry. A process for making a vegetable substitute for milk, malted nuts, was also perfected. By request of the U. S. Department of Agriculture, experiments were carried on to find a vegetable substitute for meat which resulted in the production of protose, a nut preparation, which to a considerable degree, resembles meat in appearance, taste and odor, hav-ing a slight fibre like potted meat. Some hundreds of tons of these nut foods have been made and used and they have proved to be complete nutritive substitutes for meat.

Nuts a Good Food for Nursing Mothers and Infants

The increasing incapacity of American mothers to provide lacteal nour-ishment for their infants has for years been the subject of much discussion among physicians and has come to be regarded as a just occasion for alarm as an evidence of race degeneracy and a potent cause of infant mortality.

Statistics show that the birth rate is rapidly falling in the United States as well as in all other civilized countries. At the present rate of decline no babies will be born in the year 2,000.

The American woman is for some reason losing the capacity for mother-hood. It seems that the maternal fount is drying up and with the loss of ca-pacity for feeding her offspring, the American woman is losing her fecundity. The ability to bear and to feed offspring is a physiologic unity. With failure of one function there is a corresponding decline in the other.

The Blight of the Baby Crop

There are born in this country every year 2,500,000 babies. Of these, 300,000 die before they are one year old. The mortality of bottle-fed infants is ten to twenty times as great as that of those who are breast fed. In other words, the failure of mothers to nurse their infants is responsible for the death of scores of thousands of infants annually. Every year we lose babies enough to people a large city because they are not supplied with their natu-ral food, breast milk, for which cow's milk is by no means a complete substi-tute.

A matter of such serious moment has naturally received no small amount of attention. We have a national society devoted to the "Prevention of Infant Mortality." Numerous experts have devoted much time to the study of this question. Many theories and conjectures have been presented, but few facts. Dr. Chalmers Watson of Edinburgh, some years ago made extensive feeding experiments upon rats which led him to the conclusion that the increased consumption of meat was the potent cause of the failure in the genitive power of the British race. He found that a meat diet caused in rats within two or three generations marked degeneration of the sexual glands, shriveling of the breasts and sterility. This eminent physiologist noted that in the British Islands the decline of the birth rate had been simultaneous with the marked increase in the consumption of meat within the last fifty years.

Recently, additional light has been thrown upon this subject which is of special interest to those who are concerned with dietetics.

Interesting Experiments

At the Detroit, Michigan, Woman's Hospital and Infants' Home there has recently been conducted by Dr. Hoobler an extensive series of experiments for the purpose of determining the influence of diet upon the milk production of a nursing mother. It has long been known that a simple increase of food or of fat has no other effect than to make the mother fat without increasing the flow of milk. Dr. Hoobler's experiments had for their purpose to determine the influence of individual foods and specially arranged dietaries upon the production of milk. Studies were made of the effects of meat, eggs, cow's milk, a strictly vegetable dietary (fruits, grains and vegetables), and nuts.

The influence of the diet was judged by the following points:

1. The amount of milk produced.
2. The food value of the milk.
3. The effect upon the mother as regards loss or gain of flesh.

It was found that a diet consisting largely of nuts (fifty per cent.) was far superior to any other dietary and in every particular. The amount of milk was larger than the average (14.8%), the food value was greater (30%), and the mother did better. It was noted that the mothers "took the diet readily and in fact enjoyed it." (Jour. Am. Med. Assn. Aug. 12, 1917.)

The experimenter explicitly states in his report before the American Medical Association (June, 1917), that "nut protein seems in every way as suitable for elaborating milk protein as does animal protein." This is an exceedingly important observation for it demonstrates two very interesting and basic facts:

1. That animal protein may be wholly dispensed with; that is, that a diet from which meat, milk and eggs are wholly excluded is capable of affording adequate nourishment even for a nursing mother.

2. That nuts are necessary to give completeness to a diet from which milk, meat and eggs are excluded.

The special method of research adopted by Dr. Hoobler provides a most delicate biologic test for the nutrient value of a food. The test shows the nut to be superior to meat, milk or eggs or all of these foods together in producing the highest degree of nutritive efficiency. It has heretofore been claimed that the body can make body protein more easily out of the protein of meat, milk, or eggs, that is, animal protein of some sort, than from vegetable protein. It now appears that this is not true. Nut protein is the best of all sources upon which the body may draw for its supplies of tissue building and repairing material.

Low Comparative Cost or Nuts

The high price of nuts is constantly urged as an objection to their use as a staple. It is probable that a largely increased demand would lead to so great an increase in the supply that the cost of production, and hence the cost to the consumer, would be decreased. But even at the present prices the choicest varieties of nuts are cheaper than meats if equivalent food values are compared. This is clearly shown by the following table which indicates the amounts of various flesh foods which are equivalent to one pound of walnut meats.

One pound of walnut meats equals in food value each of the following:

	Pounds
Beef loin, lean	4.00
Beef ribs, lean	6.50
Beef neck, lean	9.50
Veal	5.50
Mutton leg, lean	4.20
Ham, lean	3.00
Fowls	4.00
Chicken, broilers	10.00
Red Bass	25.00
Trout	4.80
Frogs' legs	15.00
Oysters	13.50
Lobsters	22.00
Eggs	5.00
Milk	9.50
Evaporated cream	4.00

But the great economic importance of the encouragement of nut culture in every civilized land is best shown by comparing the amount of food which may be annually produced by an acre of land planted to nut trees and the same area devoted to the production of beef. The writer is credibly informed that two acres of land and two years are required to produce a steer weighing 600 pounds. The product of one acre for one year would be one-fourth as much, or 150 pounds of steer. The same land planted to walnut trees would produce, if I am correctly informed, an average of at least 100 pounds per tree per annum for the first twenty years. Forty trees to the acre would aggregate 4,000 pounds of nuts, or 1,000 pounds of walnut meats. The highest food value which could be ascribed to the 150 pounds of beef would be

150,000 calories or food units. The food value of the nut meats would be 3,000,000 calories, or twenty times as much food from the nut trees as from the fattened steer, and food of the same general character, that is protein and fat, but of greatly superior quality.

One acre of walnut trees, 40 trees to the acre, will produce every year food equal to any one of the following items:

20,000 lbs. brook trout
5,000 lbs. beef (eight steers)
16,000 lbs. chicken broilers
34,000 lbs. lobsters
30,000 lbs. oysters
66,000 eggs (5,000 dozen)
7,000 qts. milk
A ton of mutton (13 sheep)
250,000 frogs.

And when one acre will do so much, think of the product of a million acres.

Ten times the product of all the fisheries of the country.

Half as much as all the poultry of the country.

One-seventh as much as all the beef produced.

More than twice the value of all the sheep. Half as much as all the pork. And many millions of acres may be thus utilized in nut culture.

And the walnut is not the only promising tree. The hickory, the pecan, the butternut, the filbert, and the pinon are all capable of producing equal or greater results.

A single acre of nut trees will produce protein enough to feed four persons a year and fat enough for twice that number of average persons. So 25,000,000 acres of nut trees would more than supply the whole people of the United States with their two most expensive foodstuffs. Cereals and fresh vegetables, our cheapest foods, would be needed for the carbohydrate portion of the dietary. Just think of it. A little nut orchard 200 miles square supplying one-third enough food to feed one hundred million of citizens. The trouble is the hogs and cattle are eating up our food supplies. We feed a steer 100 pounds of food and get back only 2.8 pounds. If we plant 10 pounds of corn we get back 500 pounds. If we plant one walnut we get back in twenty harvests a ton of choicest food. In nut culture there is a treasury of wealth and health and national prosperity and safety that is at present little appreciated.

Here is a veritable treasury of wealth, a potential food supply which may save the world from any suggestion of hunger for centuries to come if properly utilized.

Every man who cuts down a timber tree should be required to plant a nut tree. A nut tree has a double value. It produces valuable timber and yields every year a rich harvest of food while it is growing.

Every highway should be lined with nut trees. Nut trees will grow on land on which no other crop will grow and which is even worthless for grazing. The pinon flourishes on the bleak and barren peaks of the rockies.

The nut should no longer be considered a table luxury. It should become a staple article of food and may most profitably replace the pork and meats of various sorts which are inferior foods and are recognized as prolific sources of disease.

Ten nut trees planted for each inhabitant will insure the country against any possibility of food shortage. A row of nut trees on each side of our 3,000,000 miles of country roads will provide protein for a population of 100, 000,000. With a vanishing animal industry, nut-culture offers the only solution of the question of food supply. As the late Prof. Virchow said, "The future is with the vegetarians."

Something Must Be Done

When one contemplates the fact that the meat supply of the world is rapidly diminishing, and realizes that there is no probability that the diminished supply of animal foodstuffs will ever be materially increased but rather will steadily diminish, the importance of encouraging nut-culture will be appreciated. The human body must have for its perfect nutrition and maintenance, special proteins which appear to be found only in animal foods and nuts. To nuts, then, we must look for the future sustenance of the race. At least nuts must be used as a supplement to other vegetable foods, and in increasing quantity as the meat supply decreases.

It is certainly high time that governments, state and national, were giving attention to this highly important question. Millions of nut trees should be planted on public lands, along railroads and highways, in mountain regions and other waste places which have been denuded of their primitive forest growths. Nut pines, of which, according to Dr. Morris, there are thirty different species adapted to all conditions of climate and soil, black walnuts and hickories in the north, and in the south pecans and other subtropical nut trees, should be planted on an extensive scale. In the near future vast forests of these precious food-producing trees will be needed to supply the nutriment required by teeming millions of hungry people in this country and Europe.

Every farmer should prepare to plant a few acres of nut orchard next spring. There are millions of second growth hickories of the pignut and other worthless varieties growing in pastures and by the roadside which by grafting with shagbark cuttings may become prolific producers of one of the best of nuts.

Nut growing is certainly destined to become one of the most important of our agricultural industries. Half a century hence the nut crop will far exceed in volume and in value our present animal industry.

If the U.S. Government will secure the planting of ten nut trees for each of its 100,000,000 inhabitants, all the pastures may be converted into corn or wheat fields and all the packing houses into factories and the flocks of sheep and herds of swine and cattle may disappear, and yet no one will suffer from protein starvation.

Twenty million acres of land in walnut trees would suffice to furnish daily one-fourth of a pound of protein and half a pound of fat, the equivalent of a pound of beefsteak, and more than half a pound of butter for every man, woman and child in the republic. To what better use could we put our road-sides and a small slice of our public lands of which hundreds of millions of acres are lying waste and idle? And lands not fit for other purposes might be used for some species of nut trees.

Nuts should be eaten at every meal and made a substantial part of the bill of fare. So long as the nut is regarded as a dainty, suitable only for dessert the demand will be limited. But as its merits come to be appreciated it will be in greater demand and the industry will rapidly grow in volume. It is important, however, that the public should be educated to look upon this choicest of all nature's products as a staple food and should give to it its proper place in the national bill of fare.

The nut is the choicest aggregation of the materials essential for the building of sound human tissues, done up in a hermetically sealed package ready to be delivered by the gracious hand of Nature to those who are fortunate enough to appreciate the value of this finest of earth's bounties.

The Best Nuts

The family of edible nuts is small compared with the great variety of luscious fruits which abound in all parts of the world.

In this country, something more than a dozen excellent nuts offer, however, a sufficient variety to satisfy gustatory needs.

With two or three exceptions, nuts are rich in fat and protein and low in carbohydrates, whereas fruits, almost without exception, consist chiefly of carbohydrates, containing very little protein and almost no fats. Carbohydrates in nuts exist almost wholly in the form of sugar and dextrine, whereas in fruits we find, in addition, several varieties of acids.

Nuts are the most highly nourishing of all foodstuffs. With the exception of the chestnut, the peanut, and the litchi nut, the average nutritive value of nuts in general is about 200 calories to the ounce, or double the value of an equal quantity of starch or sugar.

Of the nuts which grow in this country, the most important are the almond, the English walnut, the pecan and the peanut. The native black walnut, the hickory nut, the pinon, the hazelnut, and the beech-nut are all valuable nuts which, by cultivation, might furnish enormous additions to our food supply. This is particularly true of the black walnut.

Among the imported nuts, the most important are the Brazil nut, the cocoanut, the pistachio, and the recently introduced litchi nut.

The Almond

This delicious nut may be placed at the head of the list as perhaps the finest of all the members of the nut family. One-fifth the weight of the almond consists of protein of the very finest quality, a larger proportion of this food element than is found in the best beefsteak, and it may be added that meat is in other respects inferior.

Besides, the almond affords more than half its weight of a most delicious and highly digestible oil, together with about one-sixth its weight of sugar, sufficient to give to it the characteristic property which gave rise to the ancient eulogistic phrase, "as sweet as a nut." Besides these rich properties, the almond contains a peculiar substance, emulsin, by the aid of which it is possible to prepare from blanched and crushed almonds, with the addition of water, a most delicious milk or cream, which, with the addition of a little sugar, very closely resembles, not only in appearance but also in nutritive properties, modified cows' milk.

The almond has the advantage over many other nuts in the fact that the astringent, leathery skin with which it is covered, may be easily removed by the simple process of blanching.

An ounce of almonds blanched and slightly roasted, or crushed and served as a nut butter, is a most wholesome addition to any meal, and may be used once or twice a day with advantage.

The Hickory Nut and the Pecan

The meat of the shellbark hickory nut is a most delicious morsel. It is richer in fat than any other nut with the exception of the pecan, a variety of the hickory which contains two-thirds its weight of easily digestible oil, with 15 per cent protein and 11 per cent carbohydrate. A pound of hickory nut meats is equal in nutritive value to more than 4 pounds of average meat. The pecan contains 4 per cent more fat and 4 per cent less protein. In food value, a pound of pecan meats exceeds the hickory nut in food value by 200 calories, and it is the most highly nutritious of all the natural products of the vegetable kingdom. In fact, with the exception of pure fat or oil, there is no food substance which offers nutritive material in so concentrated a form.

The Walnut

The native black walnut and its cousin, the butternut, are among the finest food producing trees indigenous to this country. The fat of walnut meats is nearly three-fifths, and the protein content is nearly 28 per cent, giving a nutritive value three times that of fat meat. A pound of walnuts, in fact, contains nearly 50 per cent more protein than the same quantity of beef, and two-thirds as much fat as a pound of butter. The butternut contains a little more fat than the walnut, with the same amount of protein, but barely 3 per cent of carbohydrate, less than that of any other nut, a fact which renders the butternut especially valuable for persons suffering with diabetes.

The English walnut differs from the black walnut in containing a little more fat and less than two-thirds the amount of protein. It is also slightly richer in carbohydrates. The culture of the English walnut is rapidly extending in California and recently some varieties have been produced which have proven hardy in our northern and western States, so there appears to be no reason why the English or Persian walnut may not be made to grow almost anywhere its black cousin flourishes.

The black walnut is certainly worthy of much more attention than it has received. The difficulty of removing the meat from the thick shell may be overcome by grafting ordinary stock with the newly produced thin-shelled varieties. It is claimed that a walnut tree 10 years old will produce annually 100 pounds of nuts from which 40 pounds of meats may be obtained.

Pine Nuts. — The pine nut is a seed produced in the cones of certain species of pine. More than thirty different varieties are known, varying in size from that of a lentil to a horse chestnut.

The Piñon, which grows in the western Rockies and the foothills of California, is a most delicious nut. In composition it is more than three-fifths fat and contains about two thirds as much protein as the almond. As found in the market, shelled piñons are dirty and quite unattractive in appearance, but the nut meats may be easily cleansed by washing first with ordinary water then with water containing half of one per cent of peroxide of hydrogen. This will not only cleanse but disinfect the nuts, destroying germs of any sort with which the kernels may have become infected in their peregrinations from the distant forest to the dinner table. The nut meats may be quickly dried by exposure to the heat of an oven. The flavor of the nuts is improved by very slight roasting.

The Peanut, when well dried, contains 50% more protein than the best beefsteak besides half its weight of an excellent oil.

Slightly roasted in the shell, the nut is very wholesome. The salted, roasted peanuts, however, found in the market, are often over-roasted, and on this account rather indigestible. In the form of peanut butter, first prepared by the writer nearly thirty years ago, the peanut has come to be used more extensively, perhaps, than any other nut. When properly prepared, peanut butter is easily digestible and highly nutritious. Unfortunately, many manufacturers increase their profits by using inferior and imperfect nuts. Through lack of care in roasting a certain proportion of the nuts are burned. The high temperature to which the fat is exposed produces irritating decomposition products which disturb digestion.

Instead of roasting the nuts in ordinary coffee roasters, the usual method, they should be treated by steam heat only, thus avoiding a temperature high enough to decompose the fats. Prepared in this way, nut butter is wholesome as well as palatable and a valuable addition to the diet.

The protein of the peanut has been shown by chemical research to belong to the class of complete proteins, which renders it equal to the protein of eggs and milk as a tissue-building element.

Peanuts are now largely used in the production of Malted Nuts, a substitute for milk, and Protose, a vegetable meat.

The Litchi Nut. — This nut, a native of China, which has recently been introduced into this country, is a most valuable product. It is grown in China and Honolulu, and attempts have been made through the efforts of Mr. David Fairchild, of the Agricultural Department, to introduce the cultivation of the nut in California. The nuts obtainable in our market come from China. The characteristic feature of the nut is the fact that it contains practically no fat, only a trace of protein, and nearly four-fifths its weight of carbohydrate in the form of fruit sugar, similar to the sugar of honey. It is most delicious in flavor and supplies the elements generally present only in very small proportion in other nuts.

The Cocoanut is so well known and so widely used in confections and otherwise, that scarcely anything need be said in its behalf. It should be mentioned, however, that a most excellent substitute for butter may be prepared from fresh cocoanuts by cutting the meat of the nut into strips and crushing in a meat grinder, then soaking the mass for two or three hours in several times its bulk of warm water. A rich cream will rise to the top. This is skimmed off and worked into a butter-like mass with an ordinary butter ladle. Butter prepared in this way is much used by Europeans in tropical countries.

www.ingramcontent.com/pod-product-compliance
Lightning Source LLC
Chambersburg PA
CBHW030027290326
41934CB00005B/519